Preventing Coronary Heart Disease

Editor: Amitabh Prakash

Adis International

Auckland • Buenos Aires • Chester • Hong Kong • Madrid • Milan • Osaka • Paris • Philadelphia • São Paulo • Sydney

Preventing Coronary Heart Disease

Editor: Amitabh Prakash

adis
INTERNATIONAL
A Wolters Kluwer Company

Commercial Manager: Gordon Mallarkey
Publication Manager: Lorna Venter-Lewis
Adis International Limited
 ISBN 0-86471-073-9

Earlier versions of some articles in this book were published in Adis International's peer-reviewed medical journals. The editor has collated the articles and worked with the authors to adapt and update the information for this publication.

Printed in Hong Kong.

Foreword

Coronary heart disease is a leading cause of death in developed countries. Prevention guidelines stipulate a healthy lifestyle and judicious use of drugs. However, the real foci are how to implement guidelines at a national level, how to improve outcomes, and how to select the best drug strategy.

This book contains the opinions of experts from around the world, and is designed to help you make decisions on the best way forward in preventing coronary heart disease.

Amitabh Prakash
Editor, *Drugs & Aging*

May 2000

Dr Prakash is Editor of ***Drugs & Aging****, an international journal that reviews clinical pharmacology and disease management in elderly patients. Age-related physiological changes with clinical implications for drug therapy also fall within the scope of the journal.*

Preventing Coronary Heart Disease

Contents

Guidelines for the Prevention of Coronary Heart Disease
Relating Local Needs to Local Initiatives

Ole Faergeman

Department of Medicine and Cardiology, Aarhus Amtssygehus University Hospital, Aarhus, Denmark

During the 20th century, coronary heart disease (CHD) has become the single most common cause of death in the world. In 1990, the disease caused about 12% of all deaths, and the World Health Organization expects that by the year 2020, it will be a greater burden to the national healthcare systems of the world than any other single disease.[1]

1. Guidelines for Prevention of Coronary Heart Disease (CHD)

CHD became common in the US and other western countries when inhabitants of these countries in the middle of the 20th century became increasingly physically inactive and exposed to tobacco and fat-laden food. These relationships were neither generally appreciated at first, nor was their causal nature accepted. The disease was considered preventable, treatable and possibly reversible by only a minority of medical scientists. However, evidence accumulated from basic and clinical research carried out over the last quarter century has removed most remaining scepticism concerning the possibility of prevention, and major subjects of scientific enquiry and debate now lie elsewhere.

One area, not discussed here, is the continued effort to expand our understanding of the biology of CHD on a genetic and biochemical level. Another involves the epidemiology, economics and politics of CHD, and within this area there is ongoing debate about how best to prevent this disease.

In the economically developed world, the relative risk of getting CHD has decreased until recently, almost certainly as a result of the wide adoption of better dietary habits and the decreasing use of tobacco. When the aging of populations is taken into account, however, the number of people with CHD is probably either stable or actually increasing. In the economically developing world, the incidence of CHD is rapidly increasing, partly because populations are aging everywhere and partly because of the increasing tobacco epidemic in these parts of the world.[1]

Guidelines for the prevention of CHD, based more or less on scientific evidence, have been issued by scientific societies and sometimes by health authorities in most countries of the world. In the US, the National High Blood Pressure Education Program was initiated in 1972, and since then has been regularly updated.[2] The National Cholesterol Education Program, introduced in 1986,[3,4] issued clear and far-reaching guidelines for the management of hypercholesterolaemia. In Europe, the European Atherosclerosis Society pioneered guidelines on the prevention of CHD in 1987.[5,6]

Although these guideline documents had been prepared by respected American and European scientific institutions, other institutions remained sceptical. The American College of Cardiology and the European Society of Cardiology were the most important, because cardiology is the medical specialty primarily entrusted with the diagnosis and treatment of heart disease, including CHD.

In the early 1990s, the European Society of Cardiology recognised the need to have a clearer policy on prevention. At the same time, two smaller societies, the European Atherosclerosis Society and the European Society of Hypertension, recognised that guidelines not endorsed by cardiology societies would have limited impact on clinical practice. These three societies therefore developed a set of joint guidelines; published initially in 1994,[7] they were revised in 1998.[8]

In the US, the American College of Cardiology as a first step endorsed a set of succinct, clear guidelines on secondary prevention of CHD that had been developed by the American Heart Association,[9] and the College then devoted a major conference to this issue and adopted a progressive position on the role of prevention in cardiology.[10]

2. Multiple Causes of CHD

Despite subtle differences, all of the above guidelines recognise that CHD very rarely has a single cause, as is the case in the relatively rare patients with genetically determined high levels of cholesterol in the blood (familial hypercholesterolaemia). Instead, in the majority of patients, the disease has several causes, such as moderately high hypercholesterolaemia, high blood pressure, diabetes mellitus and the smoking of tobacco. Guidelines therefore must address a complex set of issues including the identification of persons most likely to benefit from different degrees of preventive intervention and the definition of the means by which such prevention can be achieved.

Important components of such preventive efforts are well known. They include changes in lifestyle such as not smoking, avoiding obesity, and adopting a healthy diet and regular physical exercise. They also include recommendations concerning the appropriate use of drugs for the treatment of hypercholesterolaemia, high blood pressure and high blood glucose (diabetes mellitus).

3. Primary and Secondary Prevention

Guidelines virtually always include at least two strategies for the prevention of CHD; they are conventionally called primary and secondary prevention. Primary prevention embraces the measures by which healthy people can avoid getting the disease at all. Secondary prevention is the avoidance of recurrence of the disease. Both forms of prevention employ lifestyle changes and medical intervention.

4. The Scientific Basis for Guidelines

As far as possible, guidelines are based on the results of clinical science. A good example of the impact of clinical science on the formulation of guidelines is the major revision of policies and guidelines that have followed the publication of several large clinical trials the goals of which included the treatment of hypercholesterolaemia.

The Scandinavian Simvastatin Survival Study (4S) was the first of these major trials.[11] It resolved a problem that had caused much debate in the medical as well as the lay community. The problem was that some earlier clinical trials had suggested that reduction of blood cholesterol levels, while reducing myocardial infarctions, seemed to cause disease, possibly fatal, in other body systems. The 4S showed unequivocally that the overall death rate was reduced by lowering of cholesterol in patients with CHD. The reduction in deaths was due to a reduction in coronary deaths, and treatment did not cause deaths from any other condition, including cancer. Treatment also reduced the need for hospitalisations and for coronary bypass surgery. The cost effectiveness of this kind of prevention was therefore acceptable.[12,13] The results of the 4S were confirmed in later trials performed not only in patients with CHD,[14,15] but also in apparently healthy persons at high,[16] as well as low[17] risk of CHD. Placebo rates of CHD deaths per 1000 patient years were 3.8 in the West of Scotland Coronary Prevention Study (WOSCOPS)[16] and 0.9 in the Air Force/Texas Coronary Atherosclerosis Prevention Study (AFCAPS/TexCAPS).[17]

The revised position of the American College of Cardiology[9,10] was probably significantly influenced by the publication of the first of these trials,[11] and there is no question that results of clinical science in such instances influence policy, not only of medical societies, but also of government.

A major problem is that the medical literature is vast: more medical articles are published per day than is possible for one person to read in a lifetime. Methods for accumulating results of clinical research have therefore been developed,[18] ongoing clinical trials are registered systematically,[19] and strategies for developing guidelines based on systematic reviews and literature searches have been reported.[20]

In an ideal world, every element of prevention or treatment of disease should be based on good scientific evidence. In the real world, however, the value of such evidence varies substantially, and in one way or another, guideline documents can grade the firmness of the evidence on which each recommendation is based.[21] Some forms of prevention are well documented, and others are less well documented. After many years of controversy, cholesterol reduction exemplifies the former. Treatment of type 2 diabetes mellitus with insulin or oral medications exemplifies the latter. Although the risk of some of the (microvascular) complications of diabetes are lowered by reduction of blood sugar, such treatment does not improve survival.[22]

5. Typical Recommendations for CHD Prevention

The most commonly advocated recommendations for the prevention of CHD concern lifestyle changes and pharmacological intervention. Lifestyle changes are appropriate in both primary and secondary prevention, whereas drug treatment must be reserved for persons at high risk for the development of the disease and those who already have CHD.

In most guidelines, lifestyle changes involve the following:

- Diet, especially with regard to the fat composition of food. Fat should typically be restricted to less than 30% of the total energy, and guidelines usually include some kind of recommendation concerning classes of dietary fat. A typical recommendation would be that <10% of the fat should be saturated, <10% should be polyunsaturated and >10% should be monounsaturated fat. Some recommendations stipulate that food should contain less than 200 mg/day cholesterol and some emphasise the importance of eating a lot of vegetables, starchy foods, fruit and fish. The scientific basis for these recommendations is mainly a small number of clinical trials.[23-25]

- Physical exercise. A typical recommendation is 30 to 60 minutes of moderate exercise three to four times/week. These recommendations are supported by clinical trials in which exercise was a component but not the sole object of study.[26]
- Tobacco: complete cessation of consumption. The scientific basis for this recommendation is mainly physiology and observational epidemiology.

All guidelines recognise that drug treatment to prevent myocardial infarction must be reserved for persons at high risk of such an event. Patients who already have CHD typically run a 2 to 5% annual risk of recurrence of myocardial infarction and this level of risk is usually considered high enough to warrant drug therapy.

The main problem is not the patient with CHD, however. Instead, it is the assessment of risk of CHD in persons who are still apparently healthy. Guidelines differ in the way such risk is assessed. American guidelines include a number of risk factors and recommend that the decision to use drugs to lower cholesterol should depend on the level of low density lipoprotein (LDL)-cholesterol in the patient's blood and the number of other risk factors increasing that patient's risk of developing the disease.[27] The European guidelines,[7,8] and prior to them the New Zealand guidelines,[28] have employed tables giving the absolute 10-year risk of a myocardial infarction as a function of age, gender, smoking status, plasma cholesterol and systolic blood pressure. If the 10-year risk exceeds 20%, drug treatment to lower lipids and blood pressure should be considered. That would be the case, for example, if the patient is a 50-year-old male smoker with slightly elevated cholesterol and systolic blood pressure, but not if it is a woman nonsmoker of the same age, even if cholesterol and blood pressure measurements are somewhat higher.

Decisions to use lipid lowering drugs therefore become a function of a comprehensive assessment of risk. In most guidelines, decisions to use antihypertensive drugs, and especially antidiabetic drugs, depend less on such assessments, but this difference has more to do with medical orthodoxy than medical science.

Therapeutic goals vary between guidelines. In most guidelines concerning plasma lipids, goal levels are given for either cholesterol or LDL-cholesterol; some guidelines also include goals for reduction of triglycerides and increase in high-density lipoprotein (HDL) cholesterol. The goals given often depend on risk. According to the American guidelines,[9,27] for example, LDL-cholesterol should be lowered to less than 4.1 mmol/L if the person has no or only one risk factor for CHD, to less than 3.4 mmol/L if there are two or more risk factors, and to less than 2.6 mmol/L if he or she already has CHD. The new European guidelines are simpler in this respect as they recommend a goal of LDL-cholesterol <3 mmol/L for everybody, irrespective of risk. However, drugs should be used only when risk of a heart attack exceeds 20% over the next 10 years.

Guidelines concerning the management of blood pressure and blood glucose can vary similarly.

6. Conflicting Guidelines

As indicated, guidelines do not all agree, but some sets of guidelines directed at management of the same disease have been in open conflict with others. The American College of Physicians,[29] for example, issued guidelines on screening that were more conservative than and in explicit contrast to guidelines of the National Cholesterol Education Program.

In Europe, researchers in Sheffield, England, encourage a more conservative approach[30] to the management of hyperlipidaemia than do the joint European guidelines.[7,8] The disagreement is economic rather than scientific: it is that treating all persons standing to benefit from treatment according to the results of clinical trials will cost more than society can pay.

The Sheffield workers[30] have therefore proposed that drug treatment to lower cholesterol should be reserved for persons whose risk of myocardial infarction within the next 10 years exceeds 30%. In contrast, the European guidelines[7,8] call for consideration of drug therapy of high blood pressure and high cholesterol when this risk exceeds 20%. Depending on the country, this difference can encompass a large or small part of the population, and the choice of risk level can therefore also appreciably affect health resources.

The European guidelines are compatible, however, with choice of a higher risk level. In fact, health authorities could require that risk exceeds 40% before reimbursement is provided for drugs to lower cholesterol or blood pressure. Ethically untenable in this author's view, such a policy would effectively restrict use of these drugs to a very small part of the population. Thus, the European guidelines appropriately apportion responsibility for preventive care between physicians and health authorities.

7. Number Needed to Treat

The concept of 'number needed to treat' (NNT) is currently popular, because it makes decisions on important health issues apparently simple and well founded from evidence from clinical trials. If the number of patients needed to be treated with drug A for a certain period of time to prevent one heart attack or postpone one death is much higher than the number to be treated with drug B to obtain the same benefit, then obviously health authorities should fund drug B rather than drug A. Such a decision can easily be mistaken, however.

The NNT is calculated as the reciprocal of the absolute percentage difference in rates of deaths, heart attacks, etc., between the control group and the group treated with the experimental drug. For example, in the 4S trial 11.5% of control patients and 8.2% of patients treated with simvastatin died during the 5.4 years of the study. The absolute percentage difference in death rates was therefore 3.3, and it was necessary to treat 100/3.3 = 30 patients for 5.4 years with simvastatin to prevent one death. Similarly, it was necessary to treat 11 patients to prevent one heart attack.

Nonscientists are usually unaware of two major problems with the use of NNT. The first is that those who calculate NNT usually ignore the indices of statistical uncertainty that, as a matter of course, are given for the primary data.

The second is that there is no generally accepted way of selecting the data from which NNT are calculated. In some cases, NNT are based on death rates, but in others, NNT are based on rates of major or minor complications of disease. If a large number of complications are used, the absolute difference in rates between the control and the treatment group can become quite large, and NNT therefore becomes attractively but misleadingly small.[22] Moreover, NNT may not even have been based on results of clinical trials. Sometimes NNT are based entirely on observational data. For example, NNT to prevent deaths by cessation of smoking are based on observational data, because death rates were identical in the control and intervention groups of the only randomised trial of smoking cessation.[31] Based on that trial, NNT to prevent deaths by cessation of smoking therefore becomes infinite, a result rarely emphasised. Clearly, NNT are calculated in so many ways and with so many purposes that health authorities should view them very critically.

8. Relating Local Needs to Local Initiatives

Even more so than in the US, there are substantial differences within Europe in both the prevalence of coronary artery disease and in the cultural and technological background that should modify approaches to prevention as well as treatment. A recent study commissioned by the European Society of Cardiology[32] showed, for example, that the occurrence of CHD and stroke was far higher in eastern and northern Europe than in western and southern Europe. To a large extent, such differences can obviously be economically determined, but they are also influenced by national culture and politics as well as by national medical care practices. Even within an economically and culturally homogenous region of Europe such as the Nordic countries, there are important differences in disease rates and in the approaches taken by the medical community to treat and prevent the disease.[33]

The joint European guidelines[7] were therefore published as a background paper with recommendations for prevention of coronary artery disease couched in fairly general terms. The cardiology societies of Europe were asked to disseminate the joint guidelines in each country in a manner consistent with national needs.[34] The dissemination and implementation of guidelines can be encouraged by the formulation of national, or even regional, guidelines and by the organisation of shared care programmes and healthcare teams.

9. National Guidelines

National rather than international guidelines are more readily accepted by physicians for several reasons. One is that they can take into account national medical tradition and political realities such as drug reimbursement schemes. Another is that by subjecting the issue to national scrutiny and debate, guidelines pass into national ownership. This process can obviously be repeated at progressively more local levels. It is an important part of the dissemination process, because many physicians will want to satisfy themselves that guidelines issued by academic bodies are sound and consistent with their own understanding of medicine. Physicians have been trained in medical schools, which in principle are academic institutions aiming to produce graduates with independent minds and critical faculties. Such faculties can and should also be directed at guideline documents.

10. Shared Care Programmes

The term 'shared care' denotes a formalised programme for the sharing of care of the individual patient between hospital and general practice.[35] The programme is usually limited to patients with defined conditions and it defines standards of care. It does not, therefore, embrace routine communication between the two sectors of the healthcare system.

The term is new, but the concept is not. In Denmark, for example, sharing of care for pregnant women between general practitioners, midwives and hospital-based obstetricians was introduced by law in 1945 (Lov om svangerskabshygiejne). In the cardiovascular field, sharing of care is especially appropriate, either when standards of care must be very rigorous, as in anticoagulation, or when management is complex, because it includes several facets of treatment, as in secondary prevention after myocardial infarction.

Shared-care programmes can facilitate the implementation of guidelines and they lend themselves to the training of physicians and other healthcare workers. The programmes may also receive the support of the drug industry, if they encourage the wider use of particular classes of drugs.

11. Healthcare Teams

There are a large number of people either with, or at high risk for the development of, CHD, and thus the approach to prevention must be multidisciplinary. Preventive cardiology programmes should therefore involve not only cardiologists but also other specialists, such as diabetologists and general practitioners, and they must involve dieticians, nurses and often physiotherapists, occupational therapists and social workers. It therefore makes sense to organise preventive cardiology programmes as team efforts.[36]

12. Barriers to Implementation of Guidelines

CHD is common because it is brought on by the way in which we lead our lives and because there are numerous barriers to doing what we know would prevent it. Some of these barriers involve deep cultural values, best understood in anthropological terms. They include dietary traditions and norms for quality of life, such as obesity and enjoyment of tobacco as signs of wealth and wellbeing. Others are government policies such as the subsidisation of production of tobacco and foods high in animal fats, as well as reimbursement policies restricting the use of effective, but expensive, new drugs.

Within the healthcare system, important barriers to prevention are the prioritisation of acute care, time constraints, lack of skills in preventive cardiology, and many others detailed by Pearson and coworkers[10] in the report from the American College of Cardiology.

There are, however, legitimate reasons for physicians not to follow guidelines. The first has to do with the innate complexities of routine clinical practice. Opinion leaders, clinical researchers, healthcare managers and the pharmaceutical industry should recognise the differences in degrees of complexity in developing healthcare programmes or drugs for broad categories of patients on the one hand, and in dealing with individual patients on the other.

Clinical trials are experiments on humans performed under conditions as simple and well-defined as possible. Patients participating in trials should therefore not differ more from each other than necessary. To make the patient groups as homogenous as possible, clinical researchers impose restrictive criteria for inclusion and exclusion, and most patients that doctors treat in routine clinical practice would therefore not have qualified for inclusion into clinical trials. The extrapolation of results from such experiments to more complex patients, who may often be older or sick for other reasons, therefore requires clinical judgement that sometimes must result in withholding treatment that has been proven in trials to be efficacious. Good physicians do not practice 'cook book' medicine.

The second is that informed physicians may disagree with guidelines, which are not a simple function of scientific evidence. Here too, judgement is involved. Compromise and consensus are as intrinsic to the process of developing guidelines as objective evaluation and grading of scientific data, and physicians not involved in the consensus process can judge the evidence differently. Guidelines offer guidance; they are not law.

13. Closing Remarks

However well intentioned the drawing up of guidelines and the application of health economic analyses might be, both disciplines can, ironically, endanger good medical practice.

Proliferation of guidelines concerning the same clinical problem, but emanating from competing scientific societies or government agencies, can confuse physicians and provide them with an excuse for inaction. Health policies would therefore benefit from agreement between societies on the harmonisation of guidelines, when agreement is possible without compromising intellectual propriety.

As with the analyses of NNT discussed above, health economic analyses tend to be directed at new preventive interventions, based on trials providing a wealth of suitable data, rather than at well-established medical and invasive methods of treatment, which are based on less documentation and certainly on fewer data suitable for such analyses. Compared with orthodox treatments, documented new and improved ways of preventing disease are therefore disadvantaged when priorities are set by politicians and administrators.

Acknowledgement

This chapter was prepared in part during the author's tenure of grant 22511 from the Danish Heart Foundation.

References

1. Murray CJL, Lopez AD. Mortality by cause for eight regions of the world: global burden of disease study. Lancet 1997; 349: 1269-76
2. The Sixth Report of the Joint National Committee on Prevention, Detection, Evaluation, and Treatment of High Blood Pressure. Arch Intern Med 1997; 157: 2413-45
3. The Expert Panel. Report of the National Cholesterol Education Program Expert Panel on Detection, Evaluation, and Treatment of High Blood Cholesterol in Adults. Arch Intern Med 1988; 148: 36-69
4. National Cholesterol Education Program Expert Panel. Second Report of the Expert Panel on Detection, Evaluation and Treatment of High Blood Cholesterol in Adults (Adult Treatment Panel II). Circulation 1994; 89: 1329-445
5. Study Group of the European Atherosclerosis Society. Strategies for the prevention of coronary heart disease. Eur Heart J 1987; 8: 77-88
6. Study group, European Atherosclerosis Society. The recognition and management of hyperlipidaemia in adults: a policy statement of the European Atherosclerosis Society. Eur Heart J 1988; 9: 571-600
7. Pyörälä K, De Backer G, Graham I, et al. Prevention of coronary heart disease in clinical practice. Recommendations of the Task Force of the European Society of Cardiology, European Atherosclerosis Society and European Society of Hypertension. Eur Heart J 1994; 15: 1300-31
8. Wood D, De Backer G, Faergeman O, et al. Prevention of coronary heart disease in clinical practice. Eur Heart J 1998; 19: 1343-1503
9. Smith SC, Blair SN, Criqui MH, et al. Preventing heart attack and death in patients with coronary disease. Circulation 1995; 92: 2-4
10. 27th Bethesda Conference. Matching the intensity of risk factor management with the hazard for coronary disease events. J Am Coll Cardiol 1996; 27: 957-1047
11. The Scandinavian Simvastatin Survival Study Group. Randomised trial of cholesterol lowering in 4444 patients with coronary heart disease: the Scandinavian Simvastatin Survival Study (4S). Lancet 1994; 344: 1383-9
12. Jönsson B, Johannesson M, Kjekshus J, et al. Cost-effectiveness of cholesterol lowering. Eur Heart J 1996; 17: 1001-7
13. Johannesson M, Jönsson B, Kjekshus J, et al. Cost effectiveness of simvastatin treatment to lower cholesterol levels in patients with coronary heart disease. N Engl J Med 1997; 336: 332-6
14. Sacks FM, Pfeffer MA, Moye L, et al. The effect of pravastatin on coronary events after myocardial infarction in patients with average cholesterol levels. N Engl J Med 1996; 335: 1001-9

15. Long-Term Intervention with Pravastatin in Ischaemic Disease (LIPID) Study Group. Prevention of cardiovascular events and death with pravastatin in patients with coronary disease and a broad range of initial cholesterol levels. N Engl J Med 1998; 339: 1349-57
16. Shepherd J, Cobbe SM, Ford I, et al. Prevention of coronary heart disease with pravastatin in men with hypercholesterolemia. N Engl J Med 1995; 333: 1301-7
17. Downs JR, Clearfield M, Weis S, et al. Primary prevention of acute coronary events with lovastatin in men and women with average cholesterol levels. JAMA 1998; 279: 1615-22
18. Bero L, Rennie D. The Cochrane Collaboration: preparing, maintaining, and disseminating systematic reviews of the effects of health care. JAMA 1995; 27: 1993-8
19. Julian D. The Cardiovascular Clinical Trials Forum. Cardiovasc Clin Trials 1997; 1: 1-2
20. Cook DJ, Greengold NL, Ellrodt AG, et al. The relation between systematic reviews and practice guidelines. Arch Intern Med 1997; 127: 210-6
21. Sackett DL. Rules of evidence and clinical recommendations on the use of antithrombotic agents. Chest 1986; 89: 2S-3S
22. UK Prospective Diabetes Study Group. Intensive blood-glucose control with sulphonylureas or insulin compared with conventional treatment and risk of complications in patients with type 2 diabetes. Lancet 1998; 352: 837-53
23. Burr ML, Fehily AM, Gilbert JF, et al. Effects of changes in fat, fish, and fibre intakes on death and myocardial infarction. Diet and Reinfarction Trial. Lancet 1989; II: 757-61
24. Singh RB, Rastogi SS, Verma R, et al. Randomized controlled trial of cardioprotective diet in patients with recent myocardial infarction: results of one year follow up. BMJ 1992; 304: 1015-9
25. de Lorgeril M, Renaud S, Mamelle N, et al. Mediterranean alpha-linolenic acid-rich diet in secondary prevention of coronary heart disease. Lancet 1994; 343: 1454-9
26. O'Connor GT, Buring JE, Yusuf S, et al. An overview of randomized trials of rehabilitation and exercise after myocardial infarction. Circulation 1989; 80: 234-44
27. Grundy SM, Balady GJ, Criqui MH, et al. Guide to primary prevention of cardiovascular diseases. Circulation 1997; 95: 2329-31
28. Mann JI, Crooke M, Fear H, et al. Guidelines for detection and management of dyslipidaemia. N Z Med J 1993; 106: 133-41
29. American College of Physicians. Guidelines for using serum cholesterol, high-density lipoprotein cholesterol, and triglyceride levels as screening tests for preventing coronary heart disease in adult. Ann Intern Med 1996; 124: 515-7
30. Haq IU, Ramsay LE, Pickin DM, et al. Lipid-lowering for prevention of coronary heart disease: what policy now? Clin Sci 1996; 91: 399-413
31. Rose G, Hamilton PJS, Colwell L, et al. A randomised controlled trial of anti-smoking advice: 10-year results. J Epidemiol Community Health 1982; 36: 102-8
32. Sans S, Kesteloot H, Kromhout D. The burden of cardiovascular diseases mortality in Europe: Task Force of the European Society of Cardiology on Cardiovascular Mortality and Morbidity Statistics in Europe. Eur Heart J 1997; 18: 1231-48
33. Faergeman O, Kjekshus J, Cook T, et al. Differences between countries in treatment of coronary heart disease in the Scandinavian Simvastatin Survival Study (4S). Eur Heart J 1998; 19: 1531-7
34. Euroaspire Study Group. Euroaspire. A European Society of Cardiology survey of secondary prevention of coronary heart disease: principal results. Eur Heart J 1997; 18: 1569-82
35. Edwards P, Jones S, Shale D, et al. Shared care: a model for clinical management. Oxford: Radcliffe Medical Press, 1996
36. Lindsay GM, Gaw A, editors. Coronary heart disease prevention. A handbook for the health care team. New York: Churchill Livingstone, 1997

Correspondence: Dr *Ole Faergeman*, Department of Medicine and Cardiology, Aarhus Amtssygehus University Hospital, 8000 Aarhus, Denmark.
E-mail: ole.faergeman@aas.auh.dk

Optimising Outcomes in Primary Prevention of Coronary Heart Disease

Current Evidence Regarding Antihyperlipidaemic Therapy

Ivar Aursnes

Department of Pharmacotherapeutics, University of Oslo, Blindern, Oslo, Norway

Optimising outcomes when dealing with premature atherosclerosis, particularly coronary disease, starts with assessing individual risks. This is comparatively easy to do for individuals whose characteristics coincide with the characteristics of individuals already included in trials. Extrapolation to other population groups comes next. The final questions relate to an overview of how many individuals will be treated together and at what cost per gain in clinical outcome.

1. Assessing Individual Risk

1.1 A Healthy Man Aged Between 35 and 65 Years

What is the risk of a healthy male of developing premature atherosclerosis? If the man is under the age of 35 years, you can from a practical point of view disregard the risk, although this issue is debated.[1,2] If he is over 65 years, the atherosclerosis he is developing is not premature, but if he is a smoker, smoking will add considerably to his calculated risks. According to results from the Framingham investigation,[3] it will add 5 to 10 percentage points to the 5-year risk of experiencing symptoms of coronary disease, which for most individuals will mean about a doubling of the risk.

1.2 Measuring Serum Lipid Levels

Serum cholesterol level is best determined routinely or in connection with blood sampling for other blood tests. Two or more repeated measurements must be done to avoid being fooled by a phenomenon called 'regression to the mean'.[4] If serum cholesterol is above 5.2 but below 6 mmol/L, and especially if other members of his family are the same, a change in diet should be considered (fig. 1).[5] If the cholesterol level is over 7.8 mmol/L after repeated measurements and a change in diet, most probably, a lipid-lowering drug should be prescribed without further delay. If serum cholesterol lies between 6 and 7.8 mmol/L, proceed carefully in addition to changing diet.

The next step is to fully examine lipid status, which is helpful at all levels of total serum cholesterol. For that purpose a fasting blood sample is needed. Repeat the procedure and if the two tests agree, a reliable measurement of your patient's low density lipoprotein (LDL) cholesterol, high density lipoprotein (HDL) cholesterol and serum triglyceride levels will have been obtained.

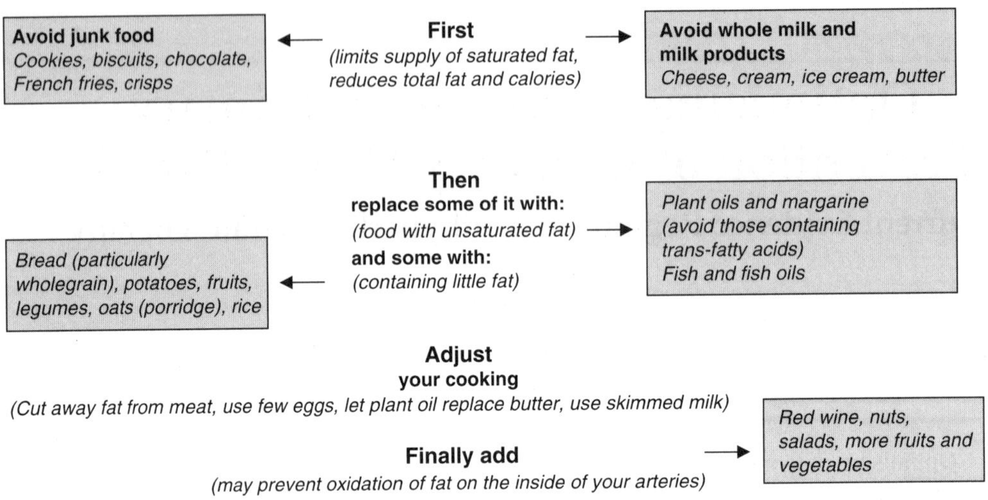

Fig. 1. A simple guide for an anticoronary change in diet.

1.3 Other Risk Factors

Suppose that total serum cholesterol level is about 7 mmol/L. That was the average level for men participating in the first clinical trial conducted that could assist with the decision whether to initiate therapy with a lipid-lowering drug or not.[6] Although the study included information about occurrence of premature atherosclerosis in the participants' families, the study's authors did not primarily include that information in the risk evaluations. As a general rule, a family history of premature coronary disease doubles the risk. Also consider whether the patient is a member of a family affected with the condition familial hypercholesterolaemia (see section 4). In addition to repeated blood pressure measurements, an ECG should also be performed to investigate whether there are signs of coronary heart disease. As a resting ECG is rather insensitive to pathology in the coronary arteries, some colleagues advocate the use of an exercise ECG in this situation. I do not follow this approach in patients totally without symptoms.

1.4 Assessing Risk

In any discussion of risk, the issue is whether your patient is a candidate for taking a lipid-lowering agent each day for years to come. In discussing this issue, the best way to formulate the risk is by stating how many individuals in the same category will have to take the drug for 5 years to avoid the risk of one of them developing serious symptoms of premature atherosclerosis. The critical number needed to treat (NNT)[7] is 33, translated from the European Guidelines.[8] This may, in your patient's view, be a too high figure for him to be interested in any regular medication. If the patient can state another number, let him do so. If he is hesitant, try to compare it with the probability of experiencing a serious accident at work during the next 5 years. What is the patient willing to do to prevent that accident? Unfortunately, one difference is that an accident may be completely avoided, whereas morbidity usually can only be delayed.

Figure 2 illustrates the results from the West of Scotland Coronary Prevention (WOSCOP) study[6] combined with data from the Framingham study (see Appendix for technical information). The risk is expressed as the critical NNT (which is the inverse of the absolute treatment effect). With this number as the basis, you can easily evaluate your patient's risk and the risk for other men between the ages of 35 and 65 years.

If the NNT is below 33 (or whatever level you agree on), the solution is to give the patient a statin (HMG-CoA reductase inhibitor). There are few adverse effects connected with such treatment.[9] In Norway, the cost may be prohibitive for some, at about $US2 per day. In case

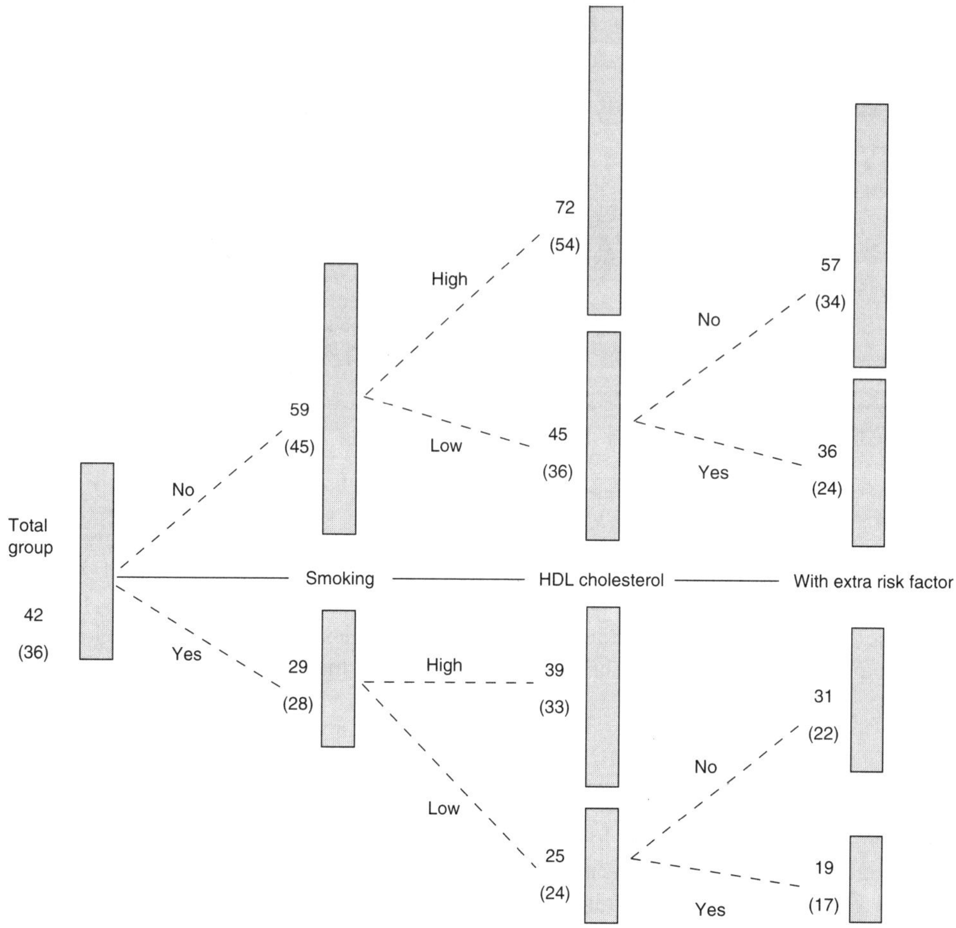

Fig. 2. Numbers needed to treat to prevent 1 coronary event during 5 years. This relates primarily to healthy men aged 35 to 65 years with total serum cholesterol level between 6.0 and 7.8 mmol/L. Based on the West of Scotland Coronary Prevention (WOSCOP) study[6] (numbers in parentheses are based on the Framingham study[3]). See Appendix for calculations.

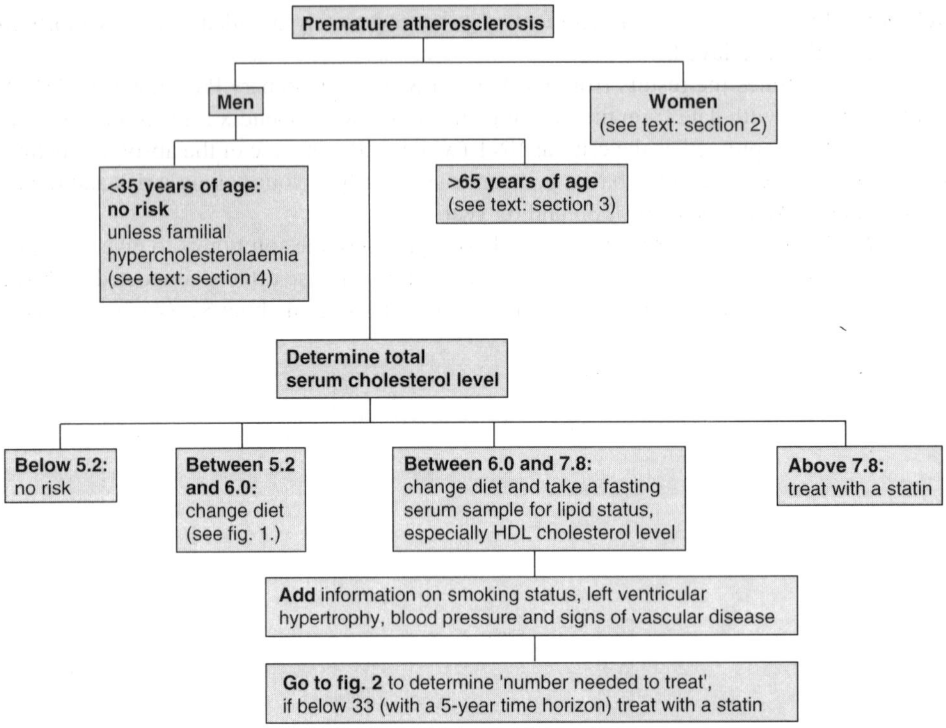

Fig. 3. Disease management algorithm for premature atherosclerosis. Figures are serum cholesterol levels in mmol/L (multiply by 38.5 to obtain mg/dl).

of insurance coverage, for instance public reimbursement of drug expenditures, my personal opinion is that it should be made effective the moment your patient shows signs of premature atherosclerosis by having disease symptoms (intermittent claudications in the legs, transitory ischaemic attacks in the brain or angina pectoris), regardless of cholesterol level. Figure 3 provides a brief outline of the described algorithm for the management of premature atherosclerosis.

2. What About Women?

There is agreement that lipid-lowering is not a 'men only' policy.[10] A popular saying is that the risk for women is the same as for men provided that they are 10 years older. An overview of cost-effectiveness studies in the field describes a consensus regarding the effect of gender. Treatment for women was found to be from 1.2 to 3.7 times more expensive than treatment for men, depending on their age.[11] It must be stressed that primary prevention studies in women are lacking. On the basis of secondary prevention studies[12,13] the effect obtained is similar to those seen in men provided the risk is the same.

The risk is very small before menopause. After that, prescription of an estrogen, in conjunction with a gestagen to prevent uterine cancer, will probably (negative so far in one study) provide a similar risk reduction to the one with statins. The risk of breast cancer is close to an odds ratio of 1 with a tendency for cancers to be more treatable in women receiving hormone replacement therapy. The latter treatment also prevents osteoporosis and takes care of vegetative symptoms connected with low estrogen levels. Later on, around the age of 60 years and over, women are definitely candidates for statin treatment, and the algorithm in figure 1 might be appropriate.

3. What About the Effect of Age?

The effect of age has been disputed. Even when a relatively narrow age span is considered, 35 to 65 years, the effects obtained and the ensuing cost effectiveness have not been agreed on. In an overview, all authors reported a U-shaped relationship, but they differed regarding the relative effect of older age as opposed to younger age.[11] In the WOSCOP study[6] (see Appendix) the NNT did not decrease with increasing age. Secondary prevention trials indicate almost unchanged effects up to 65 years of age.[12,13] For our purpose we will regard the effectiveness as unaffected by age up to 65 years. After that age we know very little but it seems reasonable to believe that the effectiveness is less in absolute terms (because atherosclerosis is due also to various other causes besides cholesterol), although the so-called 'attributable' risk is high due to high prevalence of such disease in later years. Notably, the European Guidelines,[8] by focusing on the next 10 years' absolute risk of coronary events, automatically over-emphasise the effect of age. It has been pointed out that it is illogical to use the same time frame for all age groups, and algorithms for correcting the age bias have been suggested.[14]

4. Inheritance

Most coronary patients are not members of families affected with the so-called familial hypercholesterolaemia. About 1 in 20 patients is affected, which means that they, in the heterozygotic form, have half the number of LDL receptors on cell surfaces. This increases the serum cholesterol level, mostly above 8 mmol/L, and many of the affected individuals have the characteristic tendinous xanthomas (cholesterol depositions). Each genetic mutation leading to this syndrome (worldwide almost 200) can be identified. A characteristic finding is the occurrence of one parent or child with the same disorder, as the condition is dominantly inherited. Other forms of hypercholesterolaemia are also heritable conditions, the most common one called polygenic and another named familial combined hyperlipidaemia.

From a disease management perspective, interventions should be prioritised to those with familial hypercholesterolaemia, as this condition presents itself at birth and carries a high risk. The most appropriate age to start drug therapy is debatable as it can be argued that the vascular disease process is reversible at any stage.[2]

5. Cost Effectiveness

The cost effectiveness of lipid-lowering with drugs has been extensively debated. Secondary prevention has repeatedly been shown to be highly cost effective.[15] It is understood that expenditure per life-year saved (or similar effect variables) is below, or comparable with, that of other interventions. When it comes to primary prevention there is less agreement and a wide range of figures have been reported by various authors.[11] Some of the discrepancies can be explained by different assumptions made by the different authors.

A more recent calculation of cost effectiveness has found higher costs per gain than previously reported.[16] The reasons for this discrepancy might be both differences in resources and costs included (our own endeavours have not been able to pinpoint which ones) as well as different time horizons. A time horizon of 10 years only, which is used in the most recent study, implies that while a major part of the expenditures have been included in the calculations, many benefits will occur after more than 10 years. However, as this report is easy to follow in its assumptions and its data foundation, the main findings related to primary prevention are cited in figure 4. Besides taking a conservative attitude, the main intention with that figure is to show the impact of different risks on the level of cost per life-year saved. Also, for that purpose, examples of costs of secondary prevention from the same report are included. In general, it appears that statins are priced too highly for extensive use in primary prevention.

6. The Size of the Population to be Treated

Purchasers should calculate the size of the population that will be treated before they decide on their strategy. Rather high figures were reached in doing so, as shown in figure 5 by observations from England[16] and Norway.[17] Note that while the percentages are equal for the two populations, the age distributions are dissimilar.

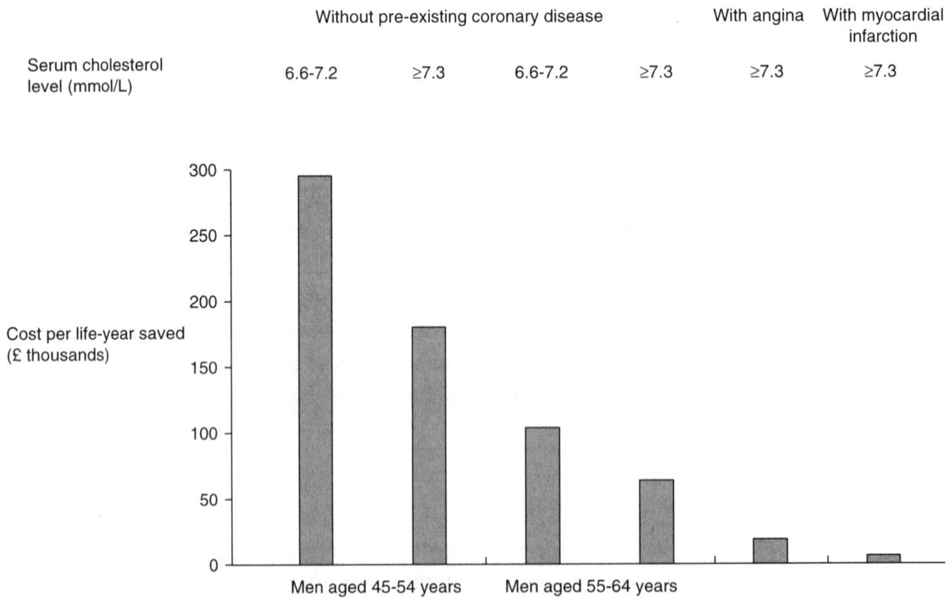

Fig. 4. Cost effectiveness of cholesterol-lowering with statins.[16]

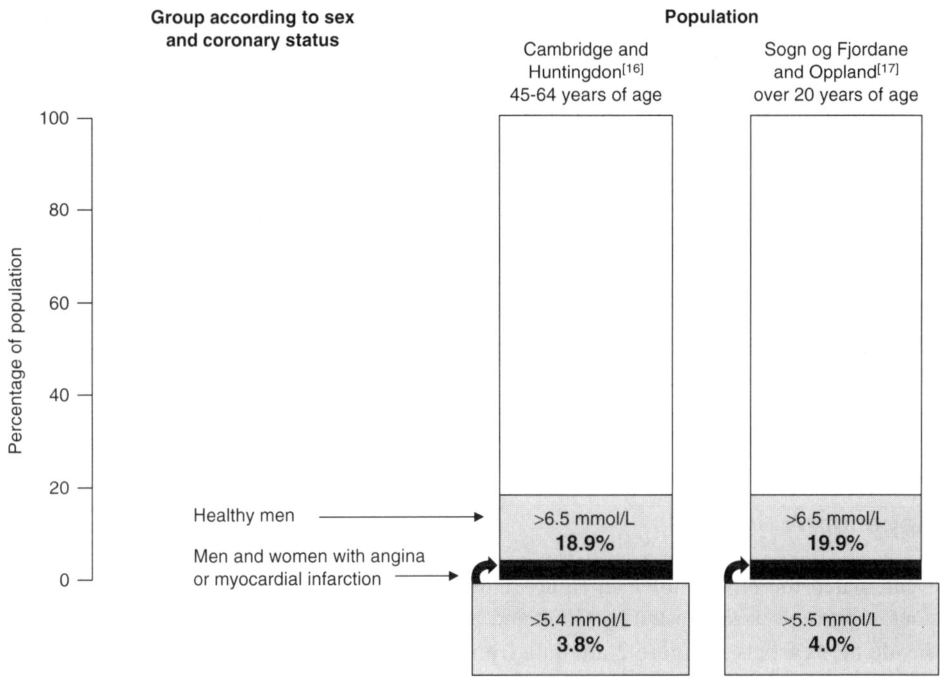

Fig. 5. The two most important subgroups (from two populations) found to be possibly qualified for lipid-lowering interventions according to gender, serum cholesterol levels (in mmol/L) and coronary status.

7. Endeavours Beyond Lipid-Lowering

After lipid-lowering there still exists a too high risk of cardiac events in the populations that have been studied.[18] Some authors and guidelines also advocate the lowering of triglycerides.[19,20] To some extent the statins take care of increased triglyceride levels and new statins are being launched that do it efficiently.[21] Another promising approach is the lowering of increased homocysteine levels with vitamin supplementations. This is suggested from a case-control analysis[22] but randomised controlled trials are lacking.

Is measuring other variables than serum cholesterol worthwhile? Apolipoproteins, especially B_{100}, Lp(a) and A_1, are interesting but thus far have been of no definite practical importance.

8. Conclusions

There is convincing evidence of the overall effect of lipid-lowering in coronary disease. Regarding primary prevention, the evidence is meagre. Regarding the reliability of the figures presented above, it is reassuring that similar results were obtained with data from two sources; a clinical trial and one with observational data. Unfortunately, as neither approach enables us to consider family history, that extra risk must be added mentally after completion of an algorithm.

It has become customary to define individuals with more than a 20% risk of a coronary event during the next 10 years as eligible for drug intervention. In terms of an NNT, with a 5-year time horizon and an expected 30% risk reduction, this will be 33. In addition, from an economical point of view, individuals with numbers less than this perhaps should be treated provided that the patient is a male between 35 and 65 years of age.

Other groups needing special consideration are women, the elderly and those with a history of coronary disease in their families. Premenopausal women will seldom be in need of drug treatment for hypercholesterolaemia. The elderly will probably be overtreated if they are subjected to the usual algorithm for total risk calculations.

The cost effectiveness of drug treatment varies considerably with the choice of patients for lipid-lowering. It is definitely too expensive for most budgets at one end of the risk distribution, while it is highly cost effective at the other. Correspondingly, the size of the population also varies considerably according to the risk level.

Appendix A

I calculated the NNT shown in figure 1 by inverting the absolute risk reductions in the various subgroups as suggested by Cook and Sackett.[7] I used 2 databases:

- Inside the brackets in figure 2 are data from the widely used Framingham equation for risk of new appearance of coronary symptoms or death.[3] In that study there was no therapeutic intervention, thus the relative risk reduction was set by me at 30% as is often done, and which is in keeping with a series of observations from interventional clinical trials.

Table I. Numbers needed to treat. Calculated from published data for relative risk reductions[6]

Variable	Subgroup	Percentage risk reduction with pravastatin (95% confidence interval)	Absolute risk reduction (%)	Numbers needed to treat	Difference between groups
Current smoking status	Nonsmoker	31 (6,48)	1.7	59	
	Smoker	31 (12,47)	3.4	29	30
HDL cholesterol level	≥43 mg/dl	33 (9,51)	1.9	52	
	<43 mg/dl	31 (11,46)	3.0	33	19
Prior vascular disease	Absent	33 (15,46)	2.3	44	
	Present	29 (−4,51)	3.2	31	13
Cholesterol level	<269 mg/dl	36 (15,51)	2.7	37	
	≥269 mg/dl	27 (4,44)	2.2	46	9
LDL cholesterol level	<189 mg/dl	37 (15,53)	2.7	37	
	≥189 mg/dl	27 (6,43)	2.2	46	9
Age	<55 years	40 (16,56)	2.6	39	
	≥55 years	27 (8,43)	2.5	40	1
Multiple risk factors	Absent	37 (20,50)	2.5	40	
	Present	20 (−13,43)	2.5	40	0

- The WOSCOP study.[6] This study is the first and only one to assess treatment effects for primary prevention of coronary disease with a statin.

I first obtained the NNT from the incidence of myocardial infarction and coronary death in the total placebo group in the WOSCOP study. The figure 7.9% minus 5.5% is inverted and gives 42. Notably, new occurrence of angina was not included as an event in the report from this study, as opposed to the Framingham data. For that reason the latter set of data should give somewhat smaller NNTs. The rest of the NNTs from the WOSCOP study[6] were derived from table I.

I omitted triglyceride levels from the table as it is well known that HDL cholesterol levels are inversely correlated with triglyceride levels. The variables are arranged in decreasing order according to differences between NNTs for the various subgroupings. Although there are wide confidence limits, the WOSCOP study data indicate that weight should be put on the variables smoking and HDL cholesterol levels (above and below 43 mg/dl or 1.1 mmol/L). This is because the relative treatment effects were the same in the subgroups made by these variables, thus producing large differences in the NNTs. The individual total cholesterol levels were all inside a narrow range, thus the effect of the cholesterol level (total and LDL) on the outcome is small. Moreover, subgrouping with or without multiple risk factors had no effect on the NNT. Also, age did not greatly influence the outcome.

The effect of combined risk factors in figure 1 was calculated by multiplication of the individual effects in the subgroups. As an example: the absolute risk connected with smoking is 10.4%, corresponding to a relative risk of 10.4/7.9, and risks with low HDL cholesterol level was an absolute risk of 9.7% and a relative risk of 9.7/7.9. The combined relative risk is by multiplication $10.4 \times 9.7/7.9^2$ and the absolute combined risk, after multiplication with risk in the whole placebo group, is $10.4 \times 9.7/7.9 = 12.8$. A treatment effect of a 32% reduction in events is calculated as the average of the effects in smokers (33%) and in individuals with low HDL cholesterol (31%), giving a absolute treatment effect of $32\% \times 12.8\% = 4.0\%$. By inversion, I obtained 25 patients needed to treat in figure 1 (this procedure is not entirely without model assumptions. Adding the effects, alternatively, did not make much difference: combined percentage risk $10.4 - 7.9 + 9.7 - 7.9 + 7.9 = 12.2$, treatment effect 3.9% and NNT = 26).

As a pragmatic solution I added to the algorithm the effect, in a hypothetical subgroup, of reducing a 5-year risk from 10% to 7%, as opposed to the whole group mean of 7.9%. This can also be used, alternatively, for the presence of hypertension (data not explicitly reported from WOSCOP), concurrent signs of vascular disease or a coexistence of several minor risk factors. It can also be used for 'coronary disease in the family', a diagnosis of familial hypercholesterolaemia (see section 4) implying even higher risk.

To calculate the corresponding figures from the Framingham data, the mean value of the highest and lowest halves of the WOSCOP risk variable level distributions (67% of a standard deviation above and below the total mean) were in sequence fed into the Framingham equation.[3] Diabetes was set to zero as well as signs of left ventricular hypertrophy. The effects of smoking and of high versus low HDL cholesterol levels were inserted in various combinations. I used the reported equation from Framingham that included the systolic (as opposed to the diastolic) blood pressure and inserted the mean blood pressure value observed in WOSCOP, i.e. 136mm Hg. As an extra risk factor I subsequently inserted systolic blood pressure equal to 180mm Hg.

References

1. Forrester JS, Prediman KS. Using serum cholesterol as a screening test for preventing coronary heart disease: the five fundamental flaws of the American College of Physicians Guidelines. Am J Cardiol 1997; 79: 790-2
2. Tonstad S. A rational approach to treating hypercholesterolemia in children. Drug Saf 1997; 16: 339-41
3. Anderson KM, Wilson PW, Odell PM, et al. An updated coronary risk profile. A statement for health professionals. Circulation 1991; 83: 356-62
4. Yudkin PL, Stratton IM. How to deal with regression to the mean in intervention studies. Lancet 1996; 347: 241-3
5. Kromhout D. Diet-heart issues in pharmacological era. Lancet 1996; 348 Suppl. I: 20-2
6. Shepherd J, Cobbe SM, Ford I, et al. Prevention of coronary heart disease with pravastatin in men with hypercholesterolemia. N Engl J Med 1995; 333: 1301-7
7. Cook RJ, Sackett DL. The number needed to treat: a clinically useful measurement of treatment effect. BMJ 1995; 310: 452-4
8. Pyörälä K, De Backer G, Graham et al. Prevention of coronary heart disease in clinical practice. Recommendations of the Task Force of the European Society of Cardiology, European Atherosclerosis Society and European Society of Hypertension. Eur Heart J 1994; 15: 1300-31
9. Aursnes I. Drugs affecting lipid metabolism. In: Dukes MN, editor. Meyler's side effects of drugs. Amsterdam: Elsevier, 1996; 13: 1324-35
10. Pearson TA, Myerson M. Treatment of hypercholesterolemia in women. Equality, effectiveness, and extrapolation of evidence. JAMA 1997; 277: 1320-1
11. Thorvik E, Aursnes I, Kristiansen IS, et al. Cost-effectiveness of cholesterol-lowering drugs: a review of the evidence. Wien Klin Wochenschrift 1996; 108: 234-43
12. Scandinavian Simvastatin Survival Study Group. Randomised trial of cholesterol lowering in 4444 patients with coronary heart disease: the Scandinavian Simvastatin Survival Study (4S). Lancet 1994; 344: 1383-9
13. Sacks FM, Pfeffer MA, Moye LA, et al. The effect of pravastatin on coronary events after myocardial infarction in patients with average cholesterol levels. N Engl J Med 1996; 335: 1001-9
14. Simpson FO. Guidelines for antihypertensive therapy: problems with a strategy based on absolute cardiovascular risk. J Hypertens 1996; 14: 683-9
15. Jönsson B, Johannesson M, Kjekshus J, et al. Cost-effectiveness of cholesterol lowering. Results from the Scandinavian Simvastatin Survival Study (4S). Eur Heart J 1996; 17: 1001-7
16. Pharoah PD, Hollingworth W. Cost effectiveness of lowering cholesterol concentrations with statins in patients with and without pre-existing coronary heart disease: life table method applied to health authority population. BMJ 1996; 312: 1443-8
17. Thorvik E, Eikeland K, Stensvold I, et al. Present and future use of cholesterol-lowering drugs. In: Beermann B, Madsen S, Strandberg K, et al., editors. Treatment of hyperlipidemia. Uppsala: Medical Product Agency, 1996; (2): 147-60
18. Maher V, Sinfuego J, Chao P, et al. Primary prevention of coronary heart disease: what has WOSCOPS told us and what questions remain? Drugs 1997; 54: 1-8
19. Spencer CM, Barradell LB, Athyros VG, et al. Gemfibrozil: a reappraisal of its pharmacological properties and place in the management of dyslipidaemia. Drugs 1996; 51: 982-1018
20. Ericsson CG, Hamsten A, Nilsson J, et al. Angiographic assessment of effects of bezafibrate on progression of coronary artery disease in young male postinfarction patients. Lancet 1996; 347: 849-53
21. Dart A, Jerums G, Nicholson G, et al. A multicenter, double-blind, one-year study comparing safety and efficacy of atorvastatin versus simvastatin in patients with hypercholesterolemia. Am J Cardiol 1997; 80: 39-44
22. Graham IM, Daly LE, Refsum HM, et al. Plasma homocystein as a risk factor for vascular disease. The European Concerted Action Project. JAMA 1997; 277: 1775-81

Correspondence: Prof. *Ivar Aursnes*, Department of Pharmacotherapeutics, University of Oslo, PO Box 1065 Blindern, N-0316 Oslo, Norway.
E-mail: i.a.aursnes@ioks.uio.no

Optimising Outcomes in Secondary Prevention of Coronary Heart Disease

Current Evidence and Future Prospects

John C. LaRosa

Tulane University Medical Center, New Orleans, Louisiana, USA

Coronary disease is the leading cause of death in both men and women in developed and developing regions of the world.[1] Because atherosclerosis is a diffuse disease of arteries, it cannot be definitively treated by invasive anatomical procedures such as bypass surgery or angioplasty. The only definitive treatments for atherosclerosis are medical. This article briefly reviews such medical interventions, using guidelines developed by a consensus panel of the American Heart Association (AHA) and summarised in table I as the basis for discussion.[2] These guidelines apply to both men and women with coronary disease. A meta-analysis done subsequent to their release confirmed that such recommendations for both genders are indeed justified.[3]

1. Treatment Outcomes with Specific Interventions: Current Evidence

1.1 Smoking Cessation

There is a linear relationship between the number of cigarettes smoked and the risk of coronary disease.[4] Moreover, with smoking cessation, the risk of myocardial infarction falls almost immediately and reaches that of a nonsmoker after approximately 2 years.[5] The AHA guidelines list first, and strongly recommend, interventions leading to the complete cessation of smoking. Although it is beyond the scope of this article to review smoking cessation interventions, two issues are of particular importance.

First, while formal smoking cessation programmes are worth trying, most people who quit do so on their own. There is some evidence that women do better at smoking cessation in settings in which there is strong social support. Overall, however, no unique interventions appear to be more successful in men or women.

Second, to be successful, any intervention must involve clear and unambiguous advice from a physician that smoking is dangerous and unacceptable behaviour for anyone with coronary disease. Despite the variable rate of success, no more important intervention can be recommended.

1.2 Lipid Management

1.2.1 Benefits of Cholesterol-Lowering Interventions

Of all the risk factors for atherosclerosis, the one that is the *sine qua non* for atherogenesis is an elevated cholesterol level. In societies where average cholesterol levels are below 160 mg/dl (4.1 mmol/ L), coronary disease is uncommon, even in the presence of other risk factors such as smoking and hypertension.[6,7] Moreover, although many questions remain, there are probably more clinical trials of cholesterol lowering in patients with coronary disease than any other medical intervention. As a result of recent studies, including the Scandinavian Simvastatin Survival Study (4S),[8] the West of Scotland Coronary Prevention Study (WOSCOPS; a primary prevention study),[9] the Cholesterol and Recurrent Events (CARE) trial,[10] the Long-Term Intervention with Pravastatin Ischemic Heart Disease (LIPID) Study[11] and the Air Force/Texas Coronary Atherosclerosis Prevention Study (AFCAPS/

Table I. Guide to comprehensive risk reduction for patients with coronary and other vascular disease [based on a summary of the American Heart Association (AHA) recommendations][2]

Risk intervention	Recommendations
Smoking (goal = complete cessation)	Strongly encourage patient and family to stop smoking. Provide counselling, nicotine replacement therapy and formal cessation programmes as appropriate
Lipid management [primary goal = LDL-C <100 mg/dl (<2.6 mmol/L); secondary goals = HDL-C >35 mg/dl (>0.9 mmol/L) and TG <200 mg/dl (<2.26 mmol/L)]	Start AHA Step II Diet in all patients: ≤30% fat, <7% saturated fat, <200 mg/d cholesterol. Assess fasting lipid profile. In post-MI patients, lipid profile may take 4 to 6 weeks to stabilise. Add drug therapy according to the following guide:
	LDL-C <100 mg/dl (<2.6 mmol/L): no drug therapy
	LDL-C 100-130 mg/dl (2.6-3.4 mmol/L): consider adding drug therapy to diet[a]
	LDL-C >130 mg/dl (>3.4 mmol/L): add drug therapy to diet[a]
	HDL-C <35 mg/dl (<0.9 mmol/L): emphasise bodyweight management and physical activity. Advise smoking cessation. If needed to achieve LDL-C goals, consider niacin (nicotinic acid), statin, fibrate
Physical activity (minimum goal = 30 minutes, 3 to 4 times per week)	Assess risk, preferably with exercise test, to guide prescription. Encourage minimum of 30 to 60 minutes of moderate intensity activity 3 or 4 times weekly (walking, jogging, cycling or other aerobic activity) supplemented by an increase in daily lifestyle activities (e.g. walking breaks at work, using stairs, gardening, household work). Maximum benefit 5-6 hours a week. Advise medically supervised programmes for moderate- to high-risk patients
Bodyweight management	Start intensive diet and appropriate physical intervention, as outlined above, in patients >120% of ideal bodyweight for height. Particularly emphasise need for bodyweight loss in patients with hypertension, elevated triglycerides or elevated glucose levels
Antiplatelet agents/anticoagulants	Start aspirin (acetylsalicylic acid) 80 to 325 mg/day, if not contraindicated. Manage warfarin to international normalised ratio = 2-3.5 in post-MI patients not able to take aspirin
ACE inhibitors post-MI	Start early post-MI in stable high-risk patients (anterior MI, previous MI, Killip class II (S_3 gallop, rales, radiographic CHF). Continue indefinitely for all with LV dysfunction (ejection fraction ≤40%) or symptoms of heart failure. Use as needed to manage blood pressure or symptoms in all other patients
β-Blockers	Start in high-risk post-MI patients (arrhythmia, LV dysfunction, inducible ischaemia) at 5 to 28 days. Continue 6 months minimum. Observe usual contraindications. Use as needed to manage angina, heart rhythm, or blood pressure in all other patients
Estrogens	Consider estrogen replacement in all postmenopausal women. Individualise recommendation consistent with other health risks
Blood pressure control (goal = ≤140/90mm Hg)	Initiate lifestyle modification – bodyweight control, physical activity, alcohol moderation and moderate sodium restriction in all patients with blood pressure >140mm Hg systolic or 90mm Hg diastolic. Add blood pressure medication, individualised to other patient requirements and characteristics (i.e. age, race, need for drugs with specific benefits) if blood pressure is not less than 140mm Hg systolic or 90mm Hg diastolic in 3 months or if *initial* blood pressure is >160mm Hg systolic or 100mm Hg diastolic

a Suggested drug therapy: (i) TG <200 mg/dl (<2.26 mmol/L): statin, resin, niacin (nicotinic acid); (ii) TG 200-400 mg/dl (2.26-4.52 mmol/L): statin, niacin (nicotinic acid); (iii) TG >400 mg/dl (>4.52 mmol/L): consider combined drug therapy: niacin (nicotinic acid), fibrate, statin. If LDL-C goal not achieved, consider combination therapy.

ACE = angiotensin-converting enzyme; **CHF** = congestive heart failure; **HDL-C** = high density lipoprotein-cholesterol; **LDL-C** = low density lipoprotein-cholesterol; **MI** = myocardial infarction; **TG** = triglycerides; **LV** = left ventricular; **TG** = triglycerides.

Table II. Overall risk reduction for major coronary events by gender and age: results from major statin trials[3]

	Events/participants		Proportional risk reduction (%)	Absolute risk reduction per 1000	No. needed to treat	p-Value
	placebo	statin				
Gender						
Women	247/1968	180/194	29	33	31	<0.001
Men	1795/13429	1310/13472	31	37	27	<0.001
Age[a]						
≥ 65y	740/4508	539/4490	32	44	23	<0.001
< 65y	1302/10889	951/10930	31	32	31	<0.001

a Age > 57 years in men and > 62 years in women were used in AFCAPS/TexCAPS.

Tex CAPS; another primary prevention trial)[12] and many older studies in which cholesterol lowering was more modest, we now have unequivocal evidence that lowering low density lipoprotein cholesterol (LDL-C) can lower morbidity and mortality from subsequent coronary disease by 25 to 40%.

In meta-analysis, these studies demonstrated an overall reduction of above 30% in the relative risk of a subsequent coronary event. This effect was virtually identical in men and women, and in those under and over 65 years of age (table II). Reduction in relative risk of coronary events was slightly higher in the two primary prevention trials (34%) than in the three secondary prevention trials (30%). An overall reduction in mortality, both cardiovascular (down 27%) and total (down 21%), was also apparent.[3]

These studies demonstrate unequivocally the importance of lowering LDL-C in preventing both morbid and mortal coronary events. Some questions remain, including whether cholesterol levels lower than those achieved in these studies provide additional benefits. Nevertheless, these studies provide ample evidence that most patients at moderate to high risk of coronary events can benefit substantially from interventions to lower LDL-C.

None of these clinical trials directly addressed the issue of triglyceride lowering or of high density lipoprotein cholesterol (HDL-C) increases in those with coronary disease.

1.2.2 Benefits of Triglyceride-Lowering Interventions

No clinical trial has accrued patients primarily on the basis of their triglyceride level. Individuals with triglycerides over 300 or 400 mg/dl (3.4 to 4.5 mmol/L) have usually been excluded from cholesterol-lowering trials. Two early studies have provided some information. In the Stockholm Ischaemic Heart Disease Study,[13] the degree of triglyceride lowering, but not of total cholesterol change, was correlated with reductions in coronary mortality. In the more recent Bezafibrate Coronary Artery Intervention Trial (BECAIT), triglyceride lowering was accomplished with relatively little change in LDL-C and only modest increases in HDL C.[14] The benefit on serial coronary angiograms, however, was comparable to that seen in LDL-C lowering trials in which triglyceride lowering was minimal. The recently completed Veterans Administration High-Density Lipoprotein Intervention Trial (VA-HIT), which tested the effect of gemfibrozil on coronary patients with low HDL-C and moderately elevated triglyceride levels, demonstrated a reduction in coronary risk with increases in HDL-C and lower levels of triglyceride even though LDL-C levels remained unchanged.[15]

1.2.3 Current Treatment Recommendations

The AHA guidelines (table I) focus on LDL-C lowering because of the lack of definitive evidence for other lipid interventions.[2] These guidelines recommend that all patients with coronary atherosclerosis be placed on the Step II AHA diet, with less than 7% of calories coming from saturated fat and less than 200 mg/day of cholesterol. There is still debate concerning the length, if any, of the period of dietary intervention before cholesterol-lowering drugs are introduced in postcoronary patients.

The goal of lipid intervention is to reduce LDL-C levels to below 100 mg/dl (2.6 mmol/L). To achieve that, most patients require cholesterol-lowering treatment beyond diet. The drug of choice is usually one of the hydroxymethylglutaryl coenzyme A (HMG-CoA) reductase inhibitors ('statins'), which are potent agents for lowering LDL-C. In patients whose triglyceride levels are over 400 mg/dl (4.5 mmol/L), drugs such as nicotinic acid (niacin) or one of the fibric acid derivatives (e.g. gemfibrozil, clofibrate, bezafibrate, fenofibrate) may be added. However, care must be taken in using such combinations to watch for drug-induced myopathy. Atorvastatin, an HMG-CoA reductase inhibitor[16] which, in approved doses, has substantial LDL-C- and triglyceride-lowering properties, may obviate the need for such combinations in many patients. In any case, the use of an HMG-CoA reductase inhibitor will usually be necessary to achieve sufficient LDL-C lowering.

In patients with high triglycerides and low HDL-C, the importance of bodyweight reduction and increased physical activity is even greater, because these lipid parameters are particularly sensitive to such interventions. Again, it is important to emphasise that there are no gender differences in these recommendations, because the risk of recurrent disease in both men and women is very high and essentially equivalent.

1.3 Physical Activity and Bodyweight Management

Clinical trial evidence for the benefits of increased physical activity and decreased bodyweight are not available for either men or women. Nevertheless, the substantial effect that favourable changes in these parameters can have on lipid and blood pressure levels is a justification for intervention. Patients with coronary disease must have a formal exercise test to guide an exercise prescription. However, it is important to recognise that regular exercise can be of only moderate intensity, including such activities as walking, jogging or cycling, and still be effective. Many patients are discouraged by the thought that to derive any benefit from exercise they will be required to become the equivalent of a marathon runner.

Regular exercise is an indispensable ingredient in any bodyweight reduction programme and will enhance efforts at weight reduction. Bodyweight reduction should be prescribed for any patient with a bodyweight that is greater than 120% of ideal. Bodyweight loss can be a particularly frustrating undertaking for both patients and their physicians, particularly if a patient has been a habitual smoker. As with smoking cessation, different patients respond to different regimens, which can range from office counselling to more formalised group programmes. The importance of increased physical activity and bodyweight reduction cannot be overemphasised, not only for themselves but for their profoundly beneficial effects on other risk factors.

1.4 Restriction of Alcohol Intake

There is little question that alcohol protects against the development and expression of coronary atherosclerosis.[17] It is, however, a metabolic poison capable of directly causing cardiomyopathy, aggravating diabetes mellitus and raising blood pressure. In addition, alcohol is a highly addictive substance. For all of these reasons, recommendations to use alcohol for coronary prevention cannot be endorsed, although individual patients who are able to limit intake to very modest amounts may derive some benefit.

1.5 Pharmacological Interventions

1.5.1 Antiplatelet Agents

Treatment with aspirin (acetylsalicylic acid) or other antiplatelet agents has been shown to reduce recurrent coronary disease by approximately 25%. Meta-analyses of intervention trials with these agents in patients with occlusive vascular disease (two-thirds of whom received aspirin) have demonstrated this effect equally in men and women (fig. 1).[18] Once coronary disease has been documented, aspirin use is indicated in both men and women.

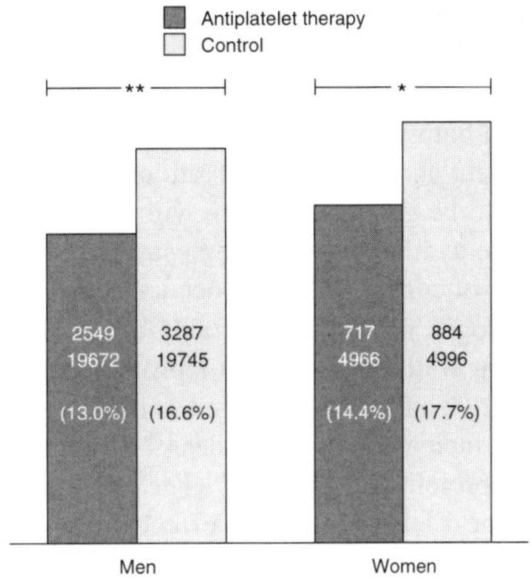

Fig. 1. The effect of antiplatelet therapy on vascular events (Antiplatelet Trialists' meta-analysis) in patients with occlusive vascular disease. Two-thirds of the patients were treated with aspirin (acetylsalicylic acid).The number of patients with events is given in each bar, followed by the total number of patients and the percentage [reproduced from Antiplatelets Trialists' Collaboration,[28] with permission).
*$p < 0.0001$; **$p < 0.00001$.

1.5.2 Angiotensin Converting Enzyme (ACE) Inhibitors

ACE inhibitors have been demonstrated in two large clinical trials to reduce both the risk of recurrent coronary disease and coronary mortality.[19,20] Patients in these studies were selected because of the presence of left ventricular dysfunction and congestive heart failure. The AHA recommends that all patients with coronary disease and who are at high risk of congestive heart failure be started on an ACE inhibitor. In those with ejection fractions of less than 40%, or with symptoms of heart failure, it is recommended that use of ACE inhibitors be continued indefinitely. Recent clinical evidence indicates that the same benefits may extend to coronary patients without heart failure.[21]

1.5.3 β-Adrenoceptor Blockers

Regular use of β-adrenoceptor blocking agents, particularly in postcoronary patients with arrhythmias, left ventricular dysfunction or recurrent ischaemia, has been demonstrated in meta-analyses to lower subsequent event rates by as much as 20 to 25%.[22] These benefits have been demonstrated most convincingly in the first year after myocardial infarction. The AHA guidelines, therefore, recommend routine use of β-adrenoceptor blockers only for the first 6 months after myocardial infarction, with the caveat that for patients with other indications, including recurrent angina, arrhythmias or hypertension, they may be continued beyond that point.

1.5.4 Estrogens

A number of observational prospective cohort studies indicate that women who report taking estrogens at any time during approximately the first 10 years after menopause have coronary and all-cause mortality rates approximately half of those in women who do not report such estrogen use.[23] More recent reports indicate that even when the estrogen is supplemented with a progestogen, benefits on coronary morbidity remain, although there are insufficient data to demonstrate effects on mortality.[24-26] These apparent benefits have been observed in women both with and without coronary disease.

Recent analyses of observational studies indicate that the potential benefit of estrogens is likely to be greatest in those with other coronary risk factors.[27,28] However, relatively few data are available concerning estrogen use in older women, in whom most of the population burden of coronary disease occurs.

Estrogen not only favourably affects lipoprotein levels but also has direct effects on the vascular wall. Favourable lipoprotein effects include an approximately 15% average decline in LDL-C, and a similar increase in HDL-C, although these effects are often accompanied by a small increase in triglycerides.[29] In addition, fibrinogen levels are decreased,[29] as are levels of lipoprotein (a) [Lp(a)].[30] The addition of a progestogen does not appear to substantially alter the LDL-C-lowering effect, although (depending on the progestogen dose) it does neutralise the HDL-C-raising effect. Benefits on fibrinogen and Lp(a) remain, although effects on the latter may be somewhat diminished.

The direct effects of estrogen on the vascular wall include inhibition of the oxidation of LDL-C as well as its uptake by the vascular wall, inhibition of platelet adhesiveness and clotting in the area of the atheroma, and the inhibition of vasospasm in the area of the atheroma. It is unclear whether or to what extent these effects are countered by progestogens. The clinical observational studies (referred to above) indicating that the addition of a progestogen to an estrogen regimen does not lower the benefit of estrogen alone, as well as animal studies indicating that the inhibition of atherogenesis by estrogen is effective even when HDL-C is lowered,[31] imply that the vascular effects of estrogens on atherogenesis may be their most important benefit and that these are relatively uninhibited by progestogens.

Only one clinical trial has formally tested the effect of hormone replacement therapy (HRT) in postmenopausal women with coronary disease. The results of that trial, the Heart and Estrogen/Progestin Replacement Study (HERS),[32] failed to demonstrate any net benefit on coronary events with a regimen of conjugated equine estrogen (0.625 and 2.5 mg/day, respectively). Whether this result would be the same if estrogen alone or in combination with another progestogen had been used is, of course, impossible to say. Nevertheless, these results should temper enthusiasm about using estrogen as a coronary preventive agent. In particular, HRT cannot be regarded as an alternative to adequate LDL-C lowering with statins or other appropriate cholesterol lowering agents.

1.5.5 Antioxidant Drugs

There has been considerable enthusiasm, based largely on observational studies in both men and women, that diets high in antioxidants such as tocopherol (vitamin E) and β-carotene appear to be associated with a lower risk of coronary disease. In a subgroup of the (all male) Physician's Health Study, β-carotene ingestion did appear to have a protective effect against coronary disease,[33] although that has not been borne out in other large clinical trials.[34,35] The notion that prescription of antioxidants is at least harmless was shaken by one trial that demonstrated that β-carotene ingestion may be associated with an increase in lung cancer in smokers.[36] At present, observational studies have not been confirmed by clinical trials of antioxidant supplementation, and the safest approach is probably to recommend diets naturally high in antioxidant vitamins rather than antioxidant supplements.

2. Control of Blood Pressure and Diabetes Mellitus

2.1 Lowering of Elevated Blood Pressure

Table III. CHD risk reduction with drug-induced BP lowering (meta-analysis of 17 trials) [after Hebert et al.[47]]

	n	Fatal	Total
Active drug	23 847	470	934
Controls	23 806	560	1104
Risk reduction (%) [95% CI]		16 (5-26)	16 (8-23)
p		0.006	0.001

BP = blood pressure; **CHD** = coronary heart disease; **CI** = confidence interval.

There is no question that control of elevated blood pressure is of substantial benefit in lowering the risk of stroke.[37] This is true of both systolic and diastolic blood pressure. The benefits of blood pressure-lowering on coronary disease predicted by observational studies have not, however, been completely supported by clinical trials. In a meta-analysis of 17 trials of drug-induced blood pressure-lowering, a 16% reduction in the risk of fatal coronary heart disease was demonstrated (table III).[37] This reduction was less than that observed in lipid-lowering trials, and less than that demonstrated in trials of β-adrenoceptor blockers or ACE inhibitors. Nevertheless, these benefits are of sufficient magnitude to justify blood pressure-lowering to prevent coronary heart disease.

Lifestyle interventions such as bodyweight reduction, salt and alcohol restriction, and regular exercise may in many cases be sufficient to bring blood pressure to acceptable levels without drug intervention. It is important to emphasise that systolic as well as diastolic blood pressure should be monitored. The evidence is now clear from the Systolic Hypertension in the Elderly Program (SHEP)[38] that treatment of elevated systolic blood pressure can reduce the incidence of stroke by 36% and the incidence of coronary heart disease by 25%.

2.2 Control of Manifestations of Diabetes Mellitus

Diabetes mellitus is a potent risk factor for the development of coronary heart disease, although this appears to be less so in populations where the intake of dietary animal fat and cholesterol is lower than in Western populations.[39] Unfortunately, there are no controlled trials of blood glucose-lowering or diabetic control to guide recommendations for coronary prevention. Clearly, lifestyle interventions such as weight loss and exercise diminish the expression of hyperglycaemia, but whether they improve the coronary risk in patients with diabetes is unknown.

Specific clinical trials of lipid lowering in patients with diabetes have not yet been reported, although the benefits in the 4S study were found in individuals both with and without diabetes.[40] Whether strict control of blood glucose, independently of any of the other risk factor modifications, is of any additional benefit in preventing expression or progression of recurrent coronary disease is also unknown. Even so, the risk of atherosclerosis is so high in patients with diabetes mellitus that lipid and glucose control regimens seem prudent, even if their benefit is not entirely certain.

3. Conclusions and Future Treatment Prospects

The definitive treatments for atherosclerosis are medical in nature. Treatment goals should include complete smoking cessation, management of lipid levels and bodyweight, regular exercise, control of blood pressure and, where indicated, intervention with antiplatelet or anticoagulant agents, ACE inhibitors, β-adrenoceptor blockers and estrogens. Failure to include these interventions in the care of patients with established coronary artery disease can be a serious and potentially life-threatening omission.

References

1. Moro CJL, Lopez AD. Mortality by cause for eight regions of the world: Global Burden of Disease Study. Lancet 1997; 349: 1269-76
2. Smith S, Blair S, Criqui MH, et al., for the Secondary Prevention Panel. Preventing heart attack deaths in patients with coronary disease. Circulation 1995; 92: 2-4
3. LaRosa JC, He J, Vupputuri S. Effect of statins on risk of coronary disease: a metaanalysis of randomized controlled trials. JAMA 1999; 282: 2340-6
4. Palmer JR, Rosenberg L, Shapiro S. 'Low yield' cigarettes and the risk of nonfatal myocardial infarction in women. N Engl J Med 1989; 320: 1569-73
5. Rosenberg L, Palmer JR, Shapiro S. Decline in the risk of myocardial infarction among women who stop smoking. N Engl J Med 1990; 322: 213-7
6. Roberts WC. Atherosclerotic risk factors: are there ten or is there only one? Am J Cardiol 1989; 64: 552-4
7. Alexander RW. Theodore Cooper Memorial Lecture. Hypertension and the pathogenesis of atherosclerosis: oxidative stress and the mediation of arterial inflammatory responses: a new perspective. Hypertension 1995; 25: 155-61
8. Scandinavian Simvastatin Survival Study Group. Randomised trial of cholesterol lowering in 4444 patients with coronary heart disease: the Scandinavian Survival Study. Lancet 1994; 344: 1383-9
9. Shepherd J, Cobbe SM, Ford I, et al. Prevention of coronary heart disease with pravastatin in men with hypercholesterolemia: West of Scotland Coronary Prevention Study Group. N Engl J Med 1995; 333: 1301-7
10. Sacks FM, Pfeffer MA, Moye LA, et al., for the Cholesterol and Recurrent Events Trial Investigators. The effect of pravastatin on coronary events after myocardial infarction in patients with average cholesterol levels. N Engl J Med 1996; 335: 1001-9
11. Long-Term Intervention with Pravastatin Ischemic Disease (LIPID) study group. Prevention of cardiovascular events and death with pravastatin in patients with coronary disease and a broad range of cholesterol levels. N Engl J Med 1998; 339: 1349-57
12. Downs JR, Clearfield M, Weis S, et al. Primary prevention of acute coronary events with lovastatin in men and women with average cholesterol levels: results of AFCAPS/Tex CAPS. JAMA 1998; 279: 1615-22
13. Carlson LA, Rosenhamer G. Reduction of mortality in the Stockholm Ischaemic Heart Disease Secondary Prevention Study by combined treatment with clofibrate and nicotinic acid. Acta Med Scand 1988; 223: 405-18
14. Ericsson CG, Hamsten A, Nilsson J, et al. Angiographic assessment of effects of bezafibrate on progression of coronary artery disease in young male postinfarction patients. Lancet 1996; 347: 849-53
15. Rubins HB, Robins SJ, Collins D, et al. Gemfibrozil for secondary prevention of coronary heart disease in men with low levels of high density lipoprotein cholesterol. N Engl J Med 1999; 341: 410-8
16. Nawrocki JW, Weiss SR, Davidson MH, et al. Reduction of LDL cholesterol by 25% to 60% in patients with primary hypercholesterolemia by atorvastatin, a new HMG-CoA reductase inhibitor. Arterioscler Thromb Vasc Biol 1995; 15: 678-82
17. Rimm EB. Klatsky A, Grobbee D, et al. Review of moderate alcohol consumption and reduced risk of coronary heart disease: is the effect due to beer, wine, or spirits? BMJ 1996; 312: 731-6
18. Antiplatelets Trialists' Collaboration. Collaborative overview of randomised trials of antiplatelet therapy: I. Prevention of death, myocardial infarction, and stroke by prolonged antiplatelet therapy in various categories of patients. BMJ 1994; 308: 81-106
19. Pfeffer MA, Braunwald E, Moye LA, et al., on behalf of the SAVE Investigators. Effect of captopril on mortality and morbidity in patients with left ventricular dysfunction after myocardial infarction: results of the survival and ventricular enlargement trial. N Engl J Med 1992; 327: 669-77
20. Yusuf A, Pepine CJ, Garces C, et al. Effect of enalapril on myocardial infarction and unstable angina in patients with low ejection fractions. Lancet 1992; 340: 1173-8
21. The Heart Outcomes Prevention Evaluation Study Investigators. Effects of an angiotensin-converting-enzyme inhibitor, ramipril, on cardiovascular events in high-risk patients. N Engl J Med 2000; 342: 145-53
22. Yusuf S, Peto R, Lewis J, et al. Beta blockade during and after myocardial infarction: an overview of randomized trials. Prog Cardiovasc Dis 1985: 27 (5): 335-71
23. Henderson BE, Pagnini-Hill A, Ross RK. Decreased mortality in users of estrogen replacement therapy. Arch Intern Med 1991; 151: 75-8
24. Falkeborn M, Persson I, Adami H-O. The risk of acute myocardial infarction after oestrogen and oestrogen-progestogen replacement. Br J Obstet Gynaecol 1992; 99: 821-8
25. Psaty BM, Heckbert SR. Atkins D, et al. The risk of myocardial infarction associated with the combination use of estrogens and progestins in postmenopausal women. Arch Intern Med 1994; 154: 1333-9
26. Grodstein F, Stampfer JJ, Manson JE, et al. Postmenopausal estrogen and progestin use and the risk of cardiovascular disease. N Engl J Med 1996; 335: 453-61
27. Girodstein F, Stampfer MJ, Colditz GA, et al. Postmenopausal hormone therapy and mortality. N Engl J Med 1997; 336: 1769-75

28. LaRosa JC. Estrogen: risk versus benefit for the prevention of coronary artery disease: review in depth. Coron Artery Dis 1993; 4: 588-94
29. Writing Group for the PEPI Trial. Effects of estrogen or estrogen/progestin regimens on heart disease risk factors in postmenopausal women: the Postmenopausal Estrogen/Progestin Interventions (PEPI) Trial. JAMA 1995; 273: 199-208
30. Kim CJ. Min YK, Ryu WS, et al. Effect of hormone replacement therapy on lipoprotein (a) and lipid levels in postmenopausal women: influence of various progestogens and duration of therapy. Arch Intern Med 1996; 156: 1693-700
31. Adams MR, Clarkson TB, Loritnik DR, et al. Contraceptive steroids and coronary artery atherosclerosis in cynomolgus macaques. Fertil Steril 1987; 47: 1010-8
32. Hulley S, Grady D, Bush, T, et al., for the Heart and Estrogen/Progestin Replacement Study (HERS) Research Group. Randomized trial of estrogen plus progestin for secondary prevention of coronary heart disease in post-menopausal women. JAMA 1998; 280: 605-13
33. Gaziano JM, Manson JE, Ridker PM, et al. Beta carotene therapy for chronic stable angina. Circulation 1991; 82 Suppl. III: 201
34. Hennekens CH, Buring JE. Manson JE, et al. Lack of effect of long-term supplementation with beta carotene on the incidence of malignant neoplasms and cardiovascular disease. N Engl J Med 1996; 334: 1145-9
35. Gaziano JM, Manson JE, Branch LG, et al. Dietary beta carotene and decreased cardiovascular mortality in an elderly cohort [abstract]. J Am Coll Cardiol 1992; 19 Suppl. A: 377A
36. Omenn GS, Goodman GE, Thornquist MD, et al. Effects of a combination of beta-carotene and vitamin A on lung cancer and cardiovascular disease. N Engl J Med 1996; 334: 1150-5
37. Hebert PR, Moser M, Mayer J, et al. Recent evidence on drug therapy of mild to moderate hypertension and decreased risk of cardiovascular heart disease. Arch Intern Med 1993; 153: 578-81
38. SHEP Cooperative Research Group. Prevention of stroke by antihypertensive drug treatment in older persons with isolated systolic hypertension: final results of the Systolic Hypertension in the Elderly Program (SHEP). JAMA 1991; 265: 3255-64
39. Ruderman NB, Schneider SH. Diabetes, exercise, and atherosclerosis. Diabetes Care 1992; 15: 1787-93
40. Pyorala K, Pedersen TR, Kjekshus J, et al., for the Scandinavian Simvastatin Survival Study (4S) Group. Cholesterol lowering with simvastatin improves prognosis of diabetic patients with coronary artery disease: a sub-group analysis of the Scandinavian Simvastatin Survival Study (4S). Diabetes Care 1997; 20: 614-20

Correspondence: *John C. LaRosa*, Tulane University Medical Center, 1430 Tulane Avenue, SL76 New Orleans, LA 70112, USA.

Coronary Heart Disease Risk Factors in the Physically Active

Impact of Exercise

Lars Bo Andersen and *Merete Hippe*

The Copenhagen Center for Prospective Population Studies, Copenhagen Hospital Corporation, Copenhagen, Denmark

During the last three decades, a great amount of evidence has been collected concerning the benefit of physical activity as protection against coronary heart disease (CHD).[1] This paper provides a brief overview of the topic.

The benefit of physical activity is achieved by different mechanisms. There is the benefit of exercise, independent of the effect on risk factors, and there are effects of exercise on risk factors such as blood lipids, blood pressure, insulin sensitivity, haemostatic factors, and obesity. Recommendations for physical activity have been given to the public in order to reduce disease, including CHD.[2,3] Even if some consensus has been reached, the mechanisms by which physical activity affects health, and the type, intensity and frequency for maximal benefit, are still matters of debate. Most agree that some physical activity is better than nothing, independent of modality.

There are several reasons why it is difficult to be specific about the exercise that provides maximal protection against CHD. In prospective studies, the patients change their physical activity habits during the follow-up; not only the amount, but also the type and intensity. Baseline intensity is a predictor of future CHD, but conclusions are not uniform.[4,5] Different types of physical activity are rarely separated into aerobic exercise, resistive exercise, etc. The study by Paffenbarger and Hale[6] is probably the only study where a resistive type of physical activity was measured primarily. Most other studies have used an index of total energy expenditure, aerobic exercise or an estimation of aerobic fitness.[7-9] In studies using fitness, the relative risk of CHD between groups is greater than in studies comparing sedentary and active groups. However, a high fitness level can be inherited along with other biological risk factors.

We do not know whether the benefit of exercise works through fitness, but a high fitness level is probably not protective in sedentary persons.[10] In some studies, a beneficial effect of an increase in physical activity or fitness level in middle-age has been found, which could suggest a causal relationship.[10-12]

Training studies, where the effect of training on CHD risk factors is measured, or cross-sectional studies analysing the associations between these variables, may not have endpoints like CHD or death. However, many of the limitations in prospective studies can be overcome. Also, physiological mechanisms responsible for the benefit of physical activity can be elucidated and important new information may be gathered from such studies. Training studies usually suffer from lack of statistical power, but the training can be very specific and maintained throughout the observation period. It is not possible to show causal relationships from cross-sectional studies, but as the number of study participants can be large, it is possible to show precise graded associations between physical parameters and CHD risk factors. Also, the beneficial effect of exercise can only be shown on the risk factors for CHD in groups where disease has not yet developed (e.g. children).

The importance of the effects of exercise on risk factors is based on the fact that lower rates of CHD have been found with lower levels of the risk factors. Atherosclerosis starts in childhood and progresses throughout life, and as a high degree of stability over time has been shown for most risk factors, it may be concluded that a low risk factor level is beneficial not only in adults, but also in children.[13-15]

In the following sections, the effects of physical activity and training on the main CHD risk factors will be reviewed. Information from cross-sectional and training studies that add to the understanding of the type, amount and intensity of exercise for maximal benefit will be emphasised.

1. Changes in Risk Factors with Exercise

1.1 Blood Pressure

Aerobic exercise lowers blood pressure in all age groups.[16,17] The effect is greater for systolic than for diastolic blood pressure, and is greater in hypertensive individuals compared with normotensive individuals.[18-21] Also, exercise reduces the risk of becoming hypertensive.[22-24] In cross-sectional studies, blood pressure is inversely related to fitness level, but in studies where both physical activity and fitness are measured, physical activity is not related to blood pressure after adjustment for fitness level.[25,26] This may be interpreted as the effect of physical activity on blood pressure being mediated through fitness.

1.2 Blood Lipids and Haemostatic Factors

There is increasing evidence that physical activity favourably influences blood lipids by an increase in high density lipoprotein level and a decrease in low density lipoprotein and triglyceride levels (table I).[27] However, there is variation between studies which may be caused by the influence of simultaneous changes in diet and bodyweight, on blood lipids and by a

Table I. Magnitude of changes in cardiovascular risk factors caused by training

Risk factor	Individuals with normal risk factor level	p-Values	High risk individuals	p-Values
Systolic blood pressure (mmHg)	↓3[18]	<0.01	↓10[1]	<0.001
Diastolic blood pressure (mmHg)	↓3[18]	<0.01	↓8[1]	<0.001
Triglycerides (mmol/L)	↓0.18[27]	<0.01	↓0.41[28] ↓0.13[29]	<0.05 NS
HDL cholesterol (mmol/L)	↑0.03[27]	NS	↑0.03[28] ↑0.04[29]	NS NS
LDL cholesterol (mmol/L)	↓0.13[27]	<0.05	↓0.13[28] ↓0.17[29]	NS NS
Total cholesterol (mmol/L)	↓0.26[27]	<0.01	↓0.04[28] ↓0.17[29]	NS NS
Insulin sensitivity (% change)	↑27[30]	<0.05	↑61-65[31]a	<0.05

a Both exercise and diet.

HDL = high density lipoprotein; **LDL** = low density lipoprotein; **NS** = not significant; ↑ indicates an increase; ↓ indicates a decrease.

mixture of acute and chronic changes in blood lipids. Changes may also be different in men and women. Most studies in men, report no change in total cholesterol and an increase in high density lipoprotein level with exercise training.[28] However, in women, exercise training seems to reduce total cholesterol.[29]

It is uncertain whether changes in blood lipids are positively related to intensity and quantity of physical activity, and to initial level of blood lipids, as is the case for blood pressure. Only a few training studies have separated individuals into those with high and low levels of blood lipids (table I). The effect of training is probably partly mediated through changes in receptors and partly through hormonal changes. Many hyperlipidaemic individuals have familial hypercholesterolaemia, which is a genetic defect, where a gene that controls the production of the lipid receptors is defective. These patients have only half the number of receptors and it may not be surprising that the effect of training in these individuals is the same as that in individuals having normal levels of lipids. However, data are still too scarce to conclude.

In addition, some studies have shown beneficial effects of physical activity on haemostatic factors (decreased fibrinogen and coagulation factor VII level and platelet adhesiveness). While there are too few studies to conclude, and not all studies are significant, most point in the same direction.[28]

1.3 Obesity

Obesity is inversely associated with activity level.[32] Exercise training improves body composition in obese individuals, however, intervention studies are rarely successful in decreasing bodyweight unless a strict diet is also followed.[33] More important than bodyweight is the fat distribution (i.e. abdominal/visceral fat) and its relationship to insulin resistance (metabolic syndrome, see section 1.5).

1.4 Smoking

Smoking is an important CHD risk factor. Physical activity and smoking are negatively related, and physically active persons are less likely to start smoking, just like smokers are more likely to drop out of exercise programmes than nonsmokers.[34,35] However, training studies have not shown changes in smoking habits.[36] The negative association between smoking and physical activity is probably due to a clustering of unhealthy habits.

1.5 Hormones

Both noradrenaline (norepinephrine) release rate, insulin sensitivity and sympathetic nervous activity are affected by training.[30] These changes are probably very important, as both increased insulin sensitivity and a lower level of noradrenaline positively affect blood pressure, blood lipids, peripheral resistance and fat storage. In fact, non–insulin-dependant diabetes mellitus is commonly associated with hypertension, and the link between these diseases is hyperinsulinaemia (metabolic syndrome).[31] Training improves tissue sensitivity to insulin. The hormonal changes are probably related to changes in maximum oxygen uptake ($\dot{V}O_{2max}$), which might suggest that fitness is a more powerful predictor of risk of CHD than physical activity itself.

2. Exercise Type, Intensity, Dose-Response and Threshold

2.1 Exercise Modality

There are improvements in many CHD risk factors with aerobic training, and trained individuals have a better risk profile compared with sedentary individuals. Even in studies using low intensity exercise, improvements have been found both in blood lipids and blood pressure. However, because of a very low initial fitness level in the individuals, improvements were also found in fitness level.[37,38] It is not possible to determine if improvements are linked to an increase in aerobic fitness level. Few studies have measured both physical activity and fitness. The relationship between CHD risk factors and physical activity disappears after adjustment for fitness level.[25,26]

In a cross-sectional study of more than 6000 17-year-olds, Andersen[39] found a negatively graded relationship between aerobic fitness and blood pressure. However, no relationship was found between the amount of sports activity and other measures of physical fitness, such as strength, muscle endurance and flexibility, and blood pressure (figs 1 and 2). Two explanations were given: (i) the use of insensitive methods, or more likely, (ii) the benefit was linked to the aerobic fitness level. Only high intensity physical activity, which is a small part of the total physical activity, would have an effect on the fitness level in a relatively fit population. These findings might suggest an upper threshold in fitness level above which no further decrease in blood pressure was found.

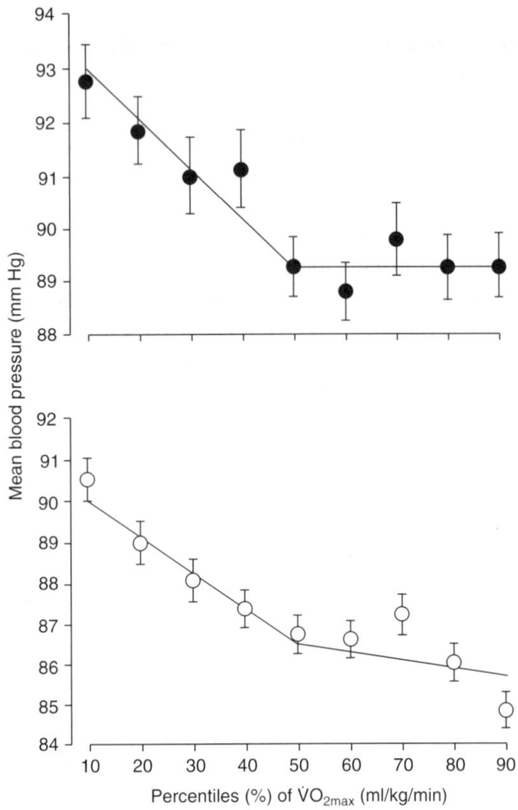

Fig. 1. Mean values and standard errors of mean for resting blood pressure in 17-year-old boys (n = 2256) **[top]** and girls (n = 3234) **[bottom]** in percentiles of maximum oxygen uptake ($\dot{V}O_{2max}$) [ml/kg/min]. The 50% percentile corresponds to 53 ml/kg/min in boys and 42 ml/kg/min in girls (reproduced from Andersen,[39] with permission).

Little evidence exists on the benefit of strength training on CHD risk factors. Several investigators have reported favourable changes in blood lipids, but data are not conclusive.[40] Kohl et al.[41] found an adverse association of muscular strength on lipid status, whereas Tucker[42] found a substantial lower risk of hypercholesterolaemia in strength-trained compared with sedentary individuals. One reason might be that strength is related to body size, and body size is also related positively to blood lipids and blood pressure. Therefore, it may be more meaningful to relate the risk factors to strength per kg bodyweight or height^2. In the study of Harris and Holly,[43] circuit weight training was found to lower blood pressure in borderline hypertensive individuals, however, an additional increase was found in aerobic fitness.[43] Compared with aerobic training, risk reductions in blood pressure and blood lipids are lower in resistive training studies, but both training modalities seem to increase insulin sensitivity.[44,45]

2.2 Intensity

Few training studies have compared the effect of different relative exercise intensities on CHD risk factors. Hicks et al.[46] found that acute changes in high density lipoprotein were positively correlated to the intensity of the exercise. However, Duncan et al.[37] found no relationship between the increase in fitness level and the increase in high density lipoprotein in three training groups walking at different speeds. The relationship may not exist, but the lack of significance could also be caused by a great daily variation in cholesterol or by changes in dietary intake with training.

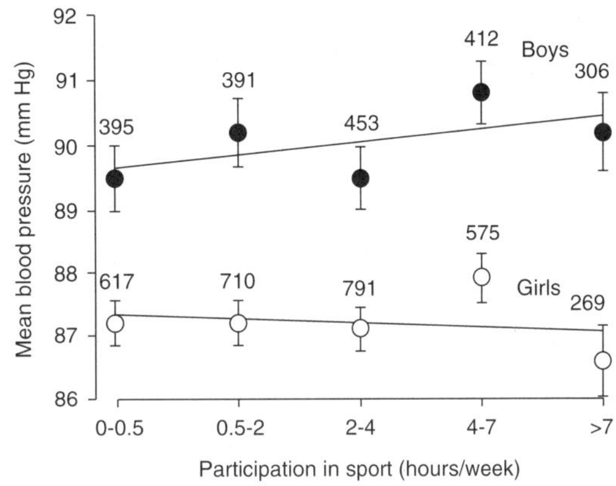

Fig. 2. Mean values and standard error of mean for blood pressure in 17-year-old boys (n = 1.957) and girls (n = 2.962) in relation to weekly hours of sports participation. The numbers above each data point represent the number of participants in each group (reproduced from Andersen,[39] with permission).

3. Future Research

Clinical exercise studies, where variations in relative intensity, total energy expenditure, exercise modality and baseline fitness level are separately controlled, are still needed before final conclusions can be drawn concerning specific recommendations of exercise for maximal benefit. Cross-sectional studies should not only be used to describe populations at risk, but also to describe relationships between variables. Also, studies of how best to motivate the population to become and remain active are needed. This is a complex task, because the type, intensity and quantity of physical activity which is good for health may change with age. The importance of the content of the physical education lessons in schools must be emphasised. In many countries, physical education lessons are compulsory and there may be a chance of motivating the sedentary if activities are chosen with care.

4. Conclusions

The benefit of being physically active is multi-faceted. There is benefit achieved independently of the effect on risk factors, and furthermore, most known CHD risk factors are favourably altered by physical activity. Part of the benefit is coupled to acute changes in risk factors, but also hormonal changes in insulin and (nor)adrenaline may play a role, as well as other changes in the cardiovascular system (more capillaries and lower peripheral resistance). Some physical activity, independent of modality, is better than none, but aerobic exercise probably alters CHD risk factors more than other types of exercise. An aerobic type of exercise sufficient to increase the fitness level may be most beneficial to CHD risk factors. However, there may be an upper level of fitness above which no further change in risk factors occurs.

References

1. Powell KE, Thompson PD, Caspersen CJ, et al. Physical activity and the incidence of coronary heart disease. Ann Rev Public Health 1987; 8: 253-87
2. Pate RR, Pratt M, Blair SN, et al. Physical activity and public health. JAMA 1995; 273: 402-7
3. Vuori I, Fentem P, Andersen LB, et al. The significance of sport for society. Counsil of Europe Press, 1995
4. Morris JN, Clayton DG, Everitt MG, et al. Exercise in leisure time: coronary attack and death rates. Br Heart J 1990; 63: 325-34
5. Wannamethee G, Shaper AG. Physical activity and stroke in British middle-aged men. BMJ 1992; 304: 601-5
6. Paffenbarger RS, Hale WE. Work activity and coronary heart mortality. N Engl J Med 1975; 292: 545-50
7. Paffenbarger RS, Hyde RT, Wing AL, et al. Physical activity, all-cause mortality, and longevity of college alumni. N Engl J Med 1986; 314: 605-13
8. Leon AS, Connett J. Physical activity and 10.5 year mortality in the Multiple Risk Factor Intervention Trial (MRFIT). Int J Epidemiol 1991; 20: 690-7
9. Blair SN, Kohl HW, Paffenbarger RS, et al. Physical fitness and all-cause mortality: a prospective study of healthy men and women. JAMA 1989; 262: 2392-401
10. Hein HO, Saudicani P, Sorensen H, et al. Changes in physical activity level and risk of ischaemic heart disease: a six year follow-up in the Copenhagen Male Study. Scand J Med Sci Sports 1994; 4: 57-64
11. Paffenbarger RS, Kampert JB, Lee I-M, et al. Changes in physical activity and other lifeway patterns influencing longevity. Med Sci Sports Exerc 1994; 26: 857-65
12. Blair SN, Kohl HW, Barlow CE, et al. Changes in physical fitness and all-cause mortality. JAMA 1995; 273: 1093-8
13. Kannel WB, Dawber TR. Atherosclerosis as a pediatric problem. J Pediatr 1972; 80: 544-54
14. Kemper HCG, Snel J, Verschuur R, et al. Tracking of health and risk indicators of cardiovascular diseases from teenager to adult: the Amsterdam Growth and Health study. Prev Med 1990; 19: 642-55
15. Andersen LB, Haraldsdottir J. Tracking of cardiovascular disease risk factors including maximal oxygen uptake and physical activity from late teenage to adulthood: an 8-year follow-up study. J Int Med Res 1993; 234: 309-15
16. Arroll B, Beaglehole R. Does physical activity lower blood pressure: a critical review of the clinical trials. J Clin Epidemiol 1992; 45: 439-47
17. Kelley G, McClellan P. Antihypertensive effects of aerobic exercise. Am J Hypertens 1994; 7: 115-9
18. Fagard RH. Prescription and results of physical activity. J Cardiovasc Pharmacol 1995; 25 Suppl. 1: s20-s27
19. Hansen HS, Froberg K, Hyldebrandt N, et al. A controlled study of eight months of physical training and reduction of blood pressure in children: the Odense schoolchild study. BMJ 1991; 303: 682-5
20. Hagberg JM, Goldring D, Ehsani AA, et al. Effect of exercise training on the blood pressure and hemodynamic features of hypertensive adolescents. Am J Cardiol 1983; 52: 763-8
21. Braith RW, Pollock ML, Lowenthal DT, et al. Moderate- and high-intensity exercise lowers blood pressure in normotensive subjects 60 to 79 years of age. Am J Cardiol 1994; 73: 1124-8
22. Gordon NF, Scott CB, Wilkinson WJ, et al. Exercise and mild essential hypertension: recommendations for adults. Sports Med 1990; 10: 390-404
23. Paffenbarger RS, Jung DL, Leung RW, et al. Physical activity and hypertension: an epidemiological view. Ann Med 1991; 23: 319-27
24. Blair SN, Goodyear NN, Gibbons LW, et al. Physical fitness and incidence of hypertension in healthy normotensive men and women. JAMA 1984; 252: 487-90
25. L¢chen M-L, Rasmussen K. The Troms¢ Study: physical fitness, self reported physical activity, and their relationship to other coronary risk factors. J Epidemiol Community Health 1992; 46: 103-7
26. Young DR, Steinhardt MA. The importance of physical fitness versus physical activity for coronary artery disease risk factors: a cross-sectional analysis. Res Q Exerc Sport 1993; 4: 377-84
27. Tran ZV, Weltman A, Glass GV, et al. The effects of exercise on blood lipids and lipoproteins: a meta-analysis of studies. Med Sci Sports Exerc 1983; 15: 393-402
28. Anderssen SA, Haaland A, Hjermann I, et al. Oslo Diet and Exercise Study: a one year randomized intervention trial; effect on haemostatic variables and other risk factors. Nutr Metab Cardiovasc Dis 1995; 5: 189-200
29. Wood PD, Haskell WL, Blair SN, et al. Increased exercise level and plasma lipoprotein concentrations: a one year, randomized, controlled study in sedentary middle-aged men. Metabolism 1983; 32: 31-9
30. Jennings G, Nelson L, Nestel P, et al. The effects of changes in physical activity on major cardiovascular risk factors, hemodynamics, sympathetic function, and glucose utilization in man: a controlled study of 4 levels of activity. Circulation 1986; 73: 30-40
31. Barnard RJ, Wen SJ. Exercise and diet in the prevention and control of the metabolic syndrome. Sports Med 1994; 18: 218-28
32. Lokey EA, Tran ZV. Effects of exercise training on serum lipid and lipoprotein concentrations in women: a meta-analysis. Int J Sports Med 1989; 10: 424-9
33. Bray GA. Exercise and obesity. In: Bouchard C, Shephard RJ, Stephens T, et al., editors. Exercise, fitness and health. Michigan: Human Kinetics Publishers, 1990: 497-510
34. Heath GW, Kendrick JS. Outrunning the risks: a behavioral risk profile of runners. Prev Med 1989; 5: 347-52
35. Marti B. Health effects of recreational running in women: some epidemiological and preventive aspects. Sports Med 1991; 11: 20-51
36. Bonanno JA, Lies JE. Effects of physical training on coronary risk factors. Am J Cardiol 1974; 33: 760-4
37. Duncan JJ, Gordon NF, Scott CB. Women walking for health and fitness. JAMA 1991; 266: 3295-9

38. Davison RCR, Grant S. Is walking sufficient exercise for health? Sports Med 1993; 16: 369-73
39. Andersen LB. Blood pressure, physical fitness and physical activity in 17-year-old Danish adolescents. J Int Med 1994; 236: 323-30
40. Kokkinos PF, Hurley BF. Strength training and lipoprotein-lipid profiles: a critical analysis and recommendations for further study. Sports Med 1990; 9: 266-72
41. Kohl HW, Gordon NF, Scott CB, et al. Musculoskeletal strength and serum lipid levels in men and women. Med Sci Sports Exerc 1992; 24: 1080-7
42. Tucker LA. Strength training and hypercholesterolemia [abstract]. Res Q Exerc Sport 1994; 65: A54-A55
43. Harris KA, Holly RG. Physiological responses to circuit weight training in borderline hypertensive subjects. Med Sci Sports Exerc 1987; 19: 246-52
44. Hurley BF. Effects of resistive training on lipoprotein-lipid profiles: a comparison to aerobic exercise training. Med Sci Sports Exerc 1989; 21: 689-93
45. Fang C-L, Sherman WM, Crouse SF, et al. Exercise modality and selected coronary risk factors: a multivariate approach. Med Sci Sports Exerc 1988; 20: 455-62
46. Hicks AL, MacDougall JD, Muckle TJ. Acute changes in high-density lipoprotein cholesterol with exercise of different intensities. J Appl Physiol 1987; 63: 1956-60

Correspondence: Dr *Lars Bo Andersen,* Institute of Preventive Medicine, Kommunehospitalet, DK-1399, Copenhagen K, Denmark.

Lipid-Lowering Treatment in Coronary Heart Disease

How Low Should Cholesterol Go?

Peter H. Jones

Associate Professor of Medicine, Section of Atherosclerosis and Lipid Research, Baylor College of Medicine, Houston, Texas, USA

Five randomised clinical trials, published since 1994, have consistently and convincingly confirmed that drug treatment to lower low-density lipoprotein cholesterol (LDL-C) levels in patients with and without manifest coronary heart disease (CHD) will significantly reduce all types of acute CHD events.[1-5] These event-based trials were preceded by a decade of lipid-lowering coronary angiographic trials, the results of which suggested that lowering LDL-C levels would delay atherosclerotic progression and, in some instances, increase the chance for regression.[6]

The combined epidemiological and trial data were carefully considered by the National Cholesterol Education Program (NCEP) Adult Treatment Panel (ATP) II and are reflected in their guidelines. These recommend drug therapy for lifestyle-resistant LDL-C levels >130 mg/dl (3.36 mmol/L) in all individuals with documented atherosclerotic vascular disease, with a target on-treatment level of ≤100 mg/dl (2.6 mmol/L).[7] For high-risk primary prevention, the LDL-C level cutpoints are ≥160 mg/dl (4.15 mmol/L) for drug therapy with a target of ≤130 mg/dl. There is no controversy about the LDL-C level treatment cutpoint for secondary prevention. However, little data exists about the clinical, or angiographic, benefits of attaining LDL-C levels well below the target level of 100 mg/dl. Additionally, other concerns have been raised about trying to achieve such an aggressive LDL-C goal. Firstly, there is one clinical end-point trial that supports a LDL-C level threshold, suggesting that reductions below 125 mg/dl (3.23 mmol/L) may not yield additional benefit.[8] Secondly, observational studies have noted possible increases in noncardiovascular disease at low cholesterol levels.[9] Finally, there are the economic considerations of potential diminishing clinical benefit as higher dosages of or combinations of drugs are used to reach lower LDL-C levels. These potentially valid concerns have confused clinicians about whether aggressive lowering of LDL-C should be pursued with single or combination drug therapy.

This chapter will focus on available epidemiological and clinical trial data that would support reducing the LDL-C below the NCEP target levels in order to maximise benefit.

1. Epidemiological Evidence of Coronary Heart Disease (CHD) Risk and Low Cholesterol Levels

The most convincing evidence that low total cholesterol levels are associated with low CHD risk comes from the 12-year follow-up of the Multiple Risk Factor Intervention Trial (MRFIT) screenees.[10] In over 350 000 individuals, the relationship between total cholesterol and CHD mortality has been shown to be curvilinear, with a continuous and graded association that extends down to a cholesterol level ≤167 mg/dl (4.3 mmol/L). The data also showed that there was no lower cholesterol threshold where CHD risk ceased to be a problem. Therefore, the lowest absolute CHD mortality occurred at total cholesterol levels of <167 mg/dl, which generally corresponds to LDL cholesterol levels at or below 100 mg/dl.

Similar to the findings in MRFIT screenees, several prospective studies have confirmed that individuals within the lowest cholesterol group have the lowest risk of CHD events. In particular, data from an 8- to 13-year prospective follow up of 9021 Chinese men and women in Shanghai concluded that death from CHD was lowest in the quartile with total cholesterol ≤3.53 mmol/L (137 mg/dl), and that no threshold existed within this low cholesterol population.[11]

In the US, it is difficult to find a significantly large number of individuals with very low cholesterol values who can be followed for sufficient time. However, the Johns Hopkins Precursor Study followed 1017 males, average age 22 years, for 30 years, and found that total cholesterol levels in young males positively and strongly predicted midlife CHD events.[12] In particular, individuals in the lowest cholesterol quartile (<172 mg/dl; 4.45 mmol/L) had not only the lowest CHD risk but the lowest total mortality as well. Therefore, observational data has consistently demonstrated that the lowest CHD risk occurs at cholesterol levels <170 mg/dl without an apparent threshold.

There was concern, however, that some observational as well as randomised treatment studies had suggested that low total cholesterol levels might be associated with an increase in noncardiovascular disease events, such as haemorrhagic stroke, cancer and suicides/accidents/trauma.[13] In particular, an National Heart, Lung and Blood Institute (NHLBI)-sponsored conference on low blood cholesterol levels concluded that observational data did support an excess of certain noncardiovascular diseases with cholesterol levels ≤160 mg/dl.[9] No unifying explanation could be formulated for the association, and the conference consensus report was unable to determine if the observation was due to confounders, competing risk or was the direct result of low cholesterol levels. Similarly, a review of three primary prevention lipid-altering trials suggested an increase in the incidence of violent deaths, such as trauma, accidents and suicide.[13]

On the other hand, a meta-analysis of published data on mortality from all causes other than CHD suggested that the only disease attributable to low cholesterol levels (especially <200 mg/dl or 5.2 mmol/L) was haemorrhagic stroke.[14] While this risk was very small, it was found only in patients with high blood pressure, and was clearly outweighed by the benefits of reduced CHD risk associated with the low cholesterol level. The authors of this analysis concluded that the association of low cholesterol levels with any noncardiovascular disease could be explained by either factors that directly caused disease (such as smoking and alcohol) or resulted from undetected disease that lowered total cholesterol levels. While the observational data on the benefit-to-risk ratio of possessing a low total cholesterol level appeared favourable, it was still not certain if drug-induced reduction of cholesterol levels was similarly free of noncardiovascular disease risk. Pending the results of the soon-to-be completed large HMG-CoA reductase inhibitor (statin) end-point trials, the prudent clinical wisdom of the early 1990s was to treat only the individuals at highest risk who had the highest LDL-C levels in order to maximise the benefit-to-risk ratio.[15]

Table I. HMG-CoA reductase inhibitor (statin) trials of low-density lipoprotein cholesterol (LDL-C) lowering: effects of treatment

Trial	Baseline LDL-C [mg/dl] (mmol/L)	Statin (mg/day)	% LDL-C change	On-treatment LDL-C [mg/dl] (mmol/L)
4S	188 (4.86)	Simvastatin 20-40	–35	122 (3.15)
CARE	139 (3.59)	Pravastatin 40	–32	98 (2.53)
LIPID	150 (3.88)	Pravastatin 40	–25	113 (2.92)
WOSCOPS	192 (4.97)	Pravastatin 40	–26	144 (3.72)
AFCAPS/TexCAPS	150 (3.88)	Lovastatin 20-40	–25	112 (2.90)

4S = The Scandinavian Simvastatin Survival Study; **AFCAPS/TexCAPS** = Air Force/Texas Coronary Atherosclerosis Prevention; Study**CARE** = Cholesterol and Recurrent Events trial; **LIPID** = Long term Intervention with Pravastatin in Ischaemic Disease study; **WOSCOPS** = West of Scotland Coronary Prevention Study.

2. Randomised Clinical Trials, CHD Events and Low Cholesterol Levels

The earliest randomised clinical trials of lipid-altering drug therapy focused on very high risk individuals with high total cholesterol and/or LDL cholesterol levels. These trials, such as the World Health Organization Clofibrate Primary Prevention Trial,[16] the Lipid Research Clinics Coronary Primary Prevention Trial,[17] the Coronary Drug Project[18] and the Helsinki Heart Study,[19] were conducted with medications that had minimal to modest effect on total cholesterol and LDL-C levels (clofibrate, cholestyramine, niacin and gemfibrozil) and/or experienced poor patient compliance at recommended dosages (cholestyramine and niacin). While some of these trials did demonstrate a reduction in CHD risk with drug treatment compared with placebo, the risk reduction was modest and no effect on total mortality was noted. More importantly, none of those trials reduced total cholesterol levels below 200 mg/dl or LDL-C levels to ≤100 mg/dl.

With the availability of the more efficacious and better tolerated statin class of drugs, five recent randomised clinical trials have shown that reductions in LDL-C levels of 25 to 35% over 5 years results in significantly lower numbers of acute coronary events, as well as lower total mortality.[1-5] The active drug treatment in these trials reduced mean LDL-C levels below 130 mg/dl in all but one [the West of Scotland Coronary Prevention Study (WOSCOPS)], and below 100 mg/dl in the Cholesterol and Recurrent Events (CARE) trial (table I). Most importantly, in each of the statin trials, there was no change in the overall incidence of any noncardiovascular event, most notably no difference in the incidence of haemorrhagic stroke, cancer or violent events. Also, simvastatin, pravastatin and lovastatin were remarkably well tolerated and free of serious adverse events. Therefore, these pivotal trials proved that potent cholesterol-lowering drug treatment of patients with more moderate hypercholesterolaemia than in earlier trials produced a greater benefit-to-risk ratio.

The question that remains to be answered is whether more aggressive lowering of LDL-C levels, particularly below the secondary prevention NCEP target of 100 mg/dl, is both well tolerated and effective. With the MRFIT screenee data as a prime example, most epidemiological studies demonstrate a curvilinear relationship between CHD risk and total cholesterol levels. The risk rapidly rises above 240 mg/dl (6.2 mmol/L), and tends to bottom out below 180 mg/dl (4.65 mmol/L). This model suggests that the predicted absolute CHD risk reduction for each incremental change (for example 30%) in LDL-C levels would be greater at the higher values than with the same incremental change in the lower values, underscoring the fact that there is diminishing incremental risk change at the lower end of the cholesterol curve (fig. 1).

This observation has led some experts to suggest that a threshold, either biological or economic, might exist at the low end of total cholesterol and/ or LDL-C levels where no further clinical benefits could be realised in primary and secondary prevention.[20] In support of this, a recent *post hoc* analysis of the CARE trial seemed to show such a threshold.[8] The incidence of cardiac events in patients with CHD randomised to pravastatin treatment for 5 years was lower across the baseline LDL-C level range of 125 to 174 mg/dl. However, individuals with baseline LDL-C levels <125mg/dl (3.2 mmol/L) had no CHD benefit with pravastatin compared with individuals receiving placebo. The authors felt that there was a LDL-C level threshold of 125 mg/dl, below which statin-induced LDL-C–lowering would offer no benefit. They concluded that while the pravastatin-treated group as a whole achieved a significant reduction in CHD events with a mean on-treatment LDL-C level of 98 mg/dl (2.5 mmol/L), the bulk of the benefit was realised in those patients whose baseline LDL-C levels were >125mg/dl.

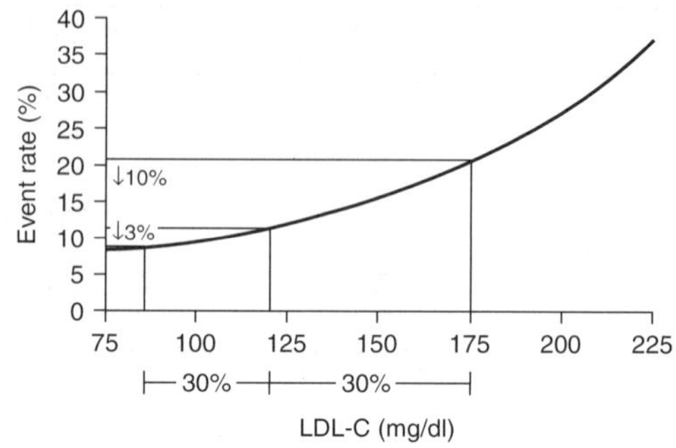

Fig. 1. Estimated incremental difference in absolute coronary heart disease event rates for a 30% decrease in low-density lipoprotein cholesterol (LDL-C), based on the Multiple Risk Factor Intervention Trial (MRFIT) Screenee data.

A similar *post hoc* analysis was performed in WOSCOPS, but with a different twist.[21] Rather than analysing the data to determine if a LDL-C level threshold existed, the authors assessed whether a 'percent LDL reduction' threshold might be operative. The majority of the CHD event reduction in pravastatin-treated CHD-free individuals occurred with only a 24% lowering from their baseline LDL-C level. Greater percentage reductions in LDL-C level and, hence, lower on-treatment LDL-C levels did not confer additional benefit. This report, therefore, suggests that in high-risk primary prevention patients with high baseline LDL-C levels, fixed-dose statin therapy produces the same risk reduction, regardless of where the baseline LDL-C starts.

Together, these two analyses would support the concept that either a modest percentage lowering of LDL-C levels is sufficient or that it is not necessary to lower LDL-C levels below 125 mg/dl in order to maximise the benefit of statin therapy in individuals at high CHD-risk.

Fortunately, there are additional lipid-lowering trials that lend support to achieving lower LDL-C treatment goals, refuting the concept of a LDL-C level benefit threshold. The Scandinavian Simvastatin Survival Study (4S) subgroup analysis evaluated the on-treatment LDL-C levels in the 2222 patients with CHD randomised to simvastatin therapy.[22] When these levels were divided into equal tertiles, there were progressively lower CHD event rates as the on-treatment LDL-C levels fell below 104 mg/dl (2.7 mmol/L). The treatment benefit was continuous but associated with progressively smaller decrements in the CHD relative risk, suggesting a curvilinear relationship. Most importantly, there was no LDL-C threshold level below 125 mg/dl.

The Long term Intervention with Pravastatin in Ischemic Disease (LIPID) trial evaluated 9014 men and women with CHD randomised to pravastatin or placebo over 6 years.[5] Analysis of treatment benefit across baseline LDL-C level tertiles of <135 mg/dl, 135 to 173 mg/dl and ≥174 mg/dl showed reduced CHD event rates in all groups. The benefit appeared to be graded, suggesting a curvilinear relative risk response to treatment. Although the mean LDL-C level in the treatment group was 113 mg/dl (2.9 mmol/L), data concerning the CHD risk reduction along the range of on-treatment LDL-C levels is not available.

In the Air Force/Texas Coronary Atherosclerosis Prevention Study (AFCAPS/TexCAPS), a similar curvilinear response was noted in the 3304 CHD-free men and women treated with lovastatin.[4] For the baseline LDL-C level tertiles of ≤142 mg/dl, 143 to 156 mg/dl and ≥157 mg/dl, lovastatin therapy for 5 years demonstrated no threshold to benefit, and the on-treatment LDL-C levels suggested progressively lower CHD events at lower LDL-C levels.

When compared with CARE and WOSCOPS, the collective 4S, LIPID and AFCAPS/TexCAPS trial results (with over 20 000 individuals) are supportive of a curvilinear relationship between LDL-C levels and CHD risk. Most importantly, these trials do not demonstrate a CHD benefit threshold when treatment to reduce LDL-C levels at or below the current NCEP target goals is pursued.

For obvious reasons, these trials evaluated statin therapy versus placebo and all clearly showed LDL-C–lowering therapy is superior to no treatment. While the majority of physicians no longer question the importance of lipid treatment, these trials did not assess the current clinical practice dilemma of whether more intensive LDL-C–lowering therapy is better than a less intensive treatment plan. To investigate this further, the Post Coronary Artery Bypass Graft (Post CABG) Trial evaluated 1351 patients with quantitative coronary angiograms over 4 years.[23] Patients were randomised to two lipid-lowering regimens; lovastatin 40 to 80 mg/day versus lovastatin 2.5 to 5 mg/day (with or without cholestyramine) in order to achieve two different on-treatment LDL-C level goals. The aggressive treatment group attained an LDL-C level of 93 to 97 mg/dl (2.4 to 2.5 mmol/L) compared with an LDL-C level of 132 to 136 mg/dl (3.4 to 3.5 mmol/ L) in the more moderate treatment group. Baseline and follow-up angiograms revealed significantly less progression in the saphenous vein grafts ($p < 0.001$), less new lesion formation ($p < 0.001$), and 29% fewer revascularisations ($p = 0.02$) in the aggressively- compared with the moderately-treated patients. In addition, analysis of treatment benefit showed that the lower on-treatment LDL-C level group had attenuation of saphenous vein graft progression regardless of the baseline high-density lipoprotein cholesterol (HDL-C) or triglyceride level.[24] This was not the case in the moderate treatment group, which demonstrated a greater progression rate with lower HDL-C and higher triglyceride values. The authors concluded that compared with moderate treatment, more aggressive LDL-C–lowering reduced atherosclerosis progression and suppressed the atherogenic potential of low HDL-C and high triglyceride levels.

Few angiographic or clinical end-point trials have been conducted with sufficient numbers of patients whose mean on-treatment LDL-C was below the 95 mg/dl level achieved in the Post-CABG study. A recently published study, the Atorvastatin versus Revascularisation Trial (AVERT), provides the first opportunity to assess the safety and clinical benefit of LDL-C–lowering substantially below 100 mg/dl in patients with CHD.[25] This unique trial evaluated stable patients with CHD and at least one significant coronary stenotic lesion who were candidates for elective angioplasty. They were randomised to receive either the indicated angioplasty (n = 177), with usual care and lipid therapy, or atorvastatin 80 mg/day (n = 164) with usual antianginal medical therapy. Follow-up was for 18 months. The primary end-point was the number of ischaemic events [CHD death, resuscitated CHD death, nonfatal myocardial infarction (MI), coronary bypass surgery, angioplasty and worsening angina pectoris requiring hospitalisation]. The lipid parameters between the two groups were significantly different in the level of LDL-C achieved: the atorvastatin treated mean LDL-C level was 77 mg/dl (2 mmol/L) [-46% reduction] and the angioplasty mean LDL-C level was 119 mg/dl (3 mmol/L) [-18% reduction]. After 18 months, 22 (13%) atorvastatin-treated patients versus 37 (21%) angioplasty patients had at least one primary end-point ($p = 0.048$; adjusted significance level was $p = 0.045$). Also, when time to first ischaemic event was analysed, the atorvastatin group had a significantly longer interval compared with the angioplasty group, with the largest differential occurring after 6 months of therapy. The atorvastatin 80 mg/day group had very few instances of significant hepatic transaminase elevations and no clinically important myositis occurred. The results of this trial confirm several important concepts. Firstly, the safety of both aggressive LDL-C–lowering well below 100 mg/dl and high-dose statin therapy are confirmed, at least for 18 months. Secondly, this degree of lipid lowering reduces the incidence of ischaemic events in as little as 6 months and is superior to a less aggressive LDL-C treatment plan. Lastly, the postulated benefit of LDL-C–lowering, which is thought to be plaque stabilisation, addresses the diffuse nature of atherosclerosis and hence affords an excellent therapy to reduce future ischaemic events which result from plaque rupture.

Several large end-point trials are in progress that should definitively answer the clinical and economic benefits, as well as the safety, of aggressive versus moderate LDL-C–lowering in patients with CHD. The first, with an expected completion in 2001, is the Study of the Effectiveness of Additional Reductions in Cholesterol and Homocysteine (SEARCH) in Great Britain. It will assess the effect of simvastatin 20 mg/day versus simvastatin 80 mg/day in 10 000 patients over a period of 5 years. The Treating to New Targets (TNT) trial is an international evaluation of atorvastatin 10 mg/day versus 80 mg/day in 10 000 patients with CHD. The study is designed to have the targeted mean LDL-C levels at approximately 100 mg/dl and 75 mg/dl (1.94 mmol/L), respectively, and will conclude when 750 primary CHD end-points occur. The Incremental Decrease in Endpoints through Aggressive Lipid-Lowering (IDEAL) trial in Scandinavia includes 7600 patients with CHD. The treatment groups are simvastatin 20 to 40 mg/day versus atorvastatin 80 mg/day. With a combined total of over 27 000 individuals, these studies should have the power to detect if there is additional benefit from high-dose statin treatment, to elucidate safety concerns and to provide data on the cost effectiveness of such statin administration.

3. Current and Future Treatment Recommendations

As discussed, the clinical trial data supports the goals of drug treatment for LDL-C levels set by the NCEP ATP II, particularly an LDL-C level ≤100 mg/dl in secondary prevention. At present, it is difficult to determine when maximal benefits of treatment have been achieved by this treatment goal. Therefore, what should the prudent clinician consider as optimal on-treatment LDL-C levels? Pending the completion of the above-mentioned trials that will test lower

Table II. Comparative dose efficacy of the statins[26]

Statin	Dose (mg)	Mean % LDL-C change
Lovastatin	20	−29
	40	−31
	80	−38
Simvastatin	10	−28
	20	−35
	40	−41
	80	−46[27]
Pravastatin	10	−19
	20	−24
	40	−34
Fluvastatin	20	−17
	40	−23
Atorvastatin	10	−38
	20	−46
	40	−51
	80	−54
Cerivastatin	0.3	−31[28]
	0.4	−36[28]

LDL-C = low-density lipoprotein cholesterol.

LDL-C level goals, the clinician should chose drug therapy to reduce LDL-C levels to 100 mg/dl. The statins are well positioned as the first-line choice for this purpose. Since there are differences in the LDL-C–lowering efficacy of the statins at various doses, the clinician should choose an appropriate starting dose that produces the desired percentage lowering of LDL-C (table II).[26] For example, a starting LDL-C level of 140 mg/dl would require a 29% reduction to reach 100 mg/dl, whereas an LDL-C level of 170 mg/dl requires a 41% reduction. If the value falls to or below 100 mg/dl, treatment should continue and no additional action on LDL-C is required. If the chosen therapy does not produce a level of 100 mg/dl, then increasing the dose of statin or initiating combination therapy [with bile-acid sequestrants or nicotinic acid (niacin)] would be required. It is important to note that when the dose of a statin is doubled, the average additional reduction in LDL-C level is about 6%. Therefore, if more than 10 to 15% additional lowering of LDL-C is required, combination therapy would be a better choice. A good example would be patients with familial hypercholesterolaemia, where combination therapy is almost always necessary to lower LDL-C levels by more than 50%. What should the clinician do if the chosen dosage of statin produces a greater than expected response and LDL-C levels fall below 70 mg/dl? Is this safe and is the benefit-to-risk ratio so favourable that no action is required? At the present time, we do not know the answer to either question. Conservative wisdom suggests reducing the dose of therapy so the LDL-C levels could increase to 100 mg/dl. On the other hand, as presented, there is no data supporting negative outcomes with a low LDL-C level and hence, a clinician with a more aggressive approach need not feel compelled to change the drug therapy. As is always the case, physician clinical judgment, considering the individual patient's history and risk factor situation as well as cost of therapy is suggested when deciding on an acceptable low-end level of LDL-C with treatment.

The ATP of the NCEP is currently meeting to evaluate all relevant data concerning lipid treatment since 1993 in order to incorporate changes in their clinical guidelines. It is anticipated that an ATP III report will be produced in 2000. One of the most important discussions will be focused on the LDL-C levels for initiation of treatment and goal cutpoints for primary and secondary prevention. I do not feel the panel will alter the secondary prevention LDL-C goal level of ≤100 mg/dl, but they may well be more supportive of clinical judgments to attain LDL-C levels closer to 80 mg/dl. For high-risk primary prevention, the LDL-C goal will still be <130 mg/dl, with the possibility of lowering the drug initiation cutpoint from 160 mg/dl to 130 mg/dl as well as supporting a more desirable goal of 100 mg/dl in certain patient subsets.

One such subset would be patients with diabetes mellitus. The American Diabetes Association has already published their own lipid treatment guidelines with a primary prevention LDL-C goal level of ≤100 mg/dl, and the ATP may well endorse that decision.[29] The AFAPS/TexCAPS results provide a rationale for considering a low HDL-C levels in men and postmenopausal women as an important identifier of high risk when LDL-C levels are >130 mg/dl. The ATP may consider drug intervention at this level for primary prevention patients with a low HDL-C level.

A unique but not uncommon dyslipidaemia, termed isolated low HDL-C, had not been addressed in previous guidelines because of little clinical trial data concerning the benefits of specific drug treatments. In the Veterans Affairs HDL Intervention Trial (VA-HIT) the patients were men with CHD whose baseline lipid profiles were: LDL-C level <130 mg/dl (mean 111 mg/dl), HDL-C level <35 mg/dl (mean 32 mg/dl) and triglyceride level <200 mg/dl (mean 162 mg/dl). There were significant reductions in recurrent nonfatal MI, CHD death and combined nonfatal MI, CHD death and stroke with gemfibrozil compared with placebo.[30] The end-point outcome was associated with a modest increase in HDL-C levels and no significant change in LDL-C levels in the gemfibrozil group. This trial the safety of fibrate drugs and that they may have an important role in secondary prevention for patients with isolated low HDL-C patients.

Finally, the ATP will address the role of borderline triglyceride levels (200 to 400 mg/dl; 5.2 to 10.3 mmol/L), with or without a concomitant elevation in LDL-C levels, with respect to modifying risk in secondary prevention. The combination of borderline triglyceride elevations and LDL-C levels ≥130 mg/dl is associated with high risk for future CHD events. Although the data are scant, the preferred treatment for this type of dyslipidaemia would be statins, since these drugs lower LDL-C levels and all apolipoprotein B-containing lipoproteins [very low density lipoproteins (VLDL), VLDL remnants and small, dense LDL particles] that may contribute to endothelial dysfunction and atherogenesis.

4. Conclusion

Several private and governmental medical practice analyses have reported that only a small minority of patients with CHD have LDL-C levels at or below 100 mg/dl. Before we can discuss how low LDL-C levels should be and whether it is safe to achieve those levels, we must first be more diligent in identifying and initiating appropriate lipid therapy in all patients with known vascular disease. Lipid-lowering treatment has proven to be one of the most effective and successful secondary prevention risk factor modifications, resulting in lower recurrent episodes of acute coronary syndromes. The marked benefit in reducing CHD death has led to improved all-cause mortality as well. The class of statin drugs has proven to be well tolerated and with good safety for this purpose, and they are considered as first-line treatment to reduce LDL-C levels. The NCEP ATPII LDL-C goal level of ≤100 mg/dl is supported by both epidemiological data, suggesting no detriment to possessing low total cholesterol and LDL-C levels, and by clinical trial data, which suggests a curvilinear reduction in CHD events as LDL-C levels approach 100 mg/dl, without an adverse effect on noncardiovascular events. How far below 100 mg/dl the LDL-C level should be driven in order to achieve as maximal an end-point benefit as possible is currently unknown. Randomised clinical trials already in progress should have the power to answer that question.

References

1. Scandinavian Simvastatin Survival Study Group. Randomized trial of cholesterol lowering 4444 patients with coronary heart disease: the Scandinavian Simvastatin Survival Study (4S). Lancet 1994; 1383-9
2. Sacks FM, Pfeffer MA, Moye LA, et al. The effect of pravastatin on coronary events after myocardial infarction in patients with average cholesterol levels. N Engl J Med 1996; 335: 1001-9
3. Shepherd J, Cobbe SM, Ford I, et al. Prevention of coronary heart disease with pravastatin in men with hypercholesterolemia. N Engl J Med 1995; 333: 1301-7
4. Downs JR, Clearfield M, Weis S, et al. Primary prevention of acute coronary events with lovastatin in men and women with average cholesterol levels: results of AFCAPS/TexCAPS. JAMA 1998; 279: 1615-22
5. The Long-Term Intervention with Pravastatin in Ishemic Disease (LIPID) Study Group. Prevention of cardiovascular events and death with pravastatin in patients with coronary heart disease and a broad range of initial cholesterol levels. N Engl J Med 1998; 339: 1349-57
6. Roussouw JE. Lipid-lowering interventions in angiographic trials. Am J Cardiol 1995; 76: 86C-92
7. National Cholesterol Education Program. Second report of the expert panel on the detection, evaluation, and treatment of high blood cholesterol in adults (Adult Treatment Panel II). Circulation 1994; 89: 1329-445
8. Sacks FM, Moye LA, Davis BR, et al. Relationship between plasma LDL concentrations during treatment with pravastatin and recurrent coronary events in the cholesterol and recurrent events trial. Circulation 1998; 97: 1446-52
9. Jacobs DR, Blackburn H, Higgins M. Report of the conference on low blood cholesterol: mortality associations. Circulation 1992; 86: 1046-60
10. Stamler J, Wentworth D, Neaton JD. Is the relationship between serum cholesterol and risk of premature death from coronary heart disease continuous and graded? Findings in 356, 222 primary screenees of the Multiple Risk Factor Intervention Trial (MRFIT). JAMA 1986; 256: 2823-8
11. Chen Z, Peto R, Collins R, et al. Serum cholesterol concentration and coronary heart disease in populations with low cholesterol concentrations. BMJ 1991; 303: 276-82
12. Klag MJ, Ford DE, Mead LA, et al. Serum cholesterol in young men and subsequent cardiovascular disease. N Engl J Med 1993; 328: 313-8
13. Muldoon MF, Manuch SB, Mathews KA. Lowering cholesterol concentrations and mortality quantitative review of primary prevention trials. BMJ 1990; 301: 309-14
14. Law MR, Thompson SG, Wald NJ. Assessing possible hazards of reducing serum cholesterol. BMJ 1994; 308: 373-9
15. Smith GD, Song F, Sheldon TA. Cholesterol lowering and mortality: the importance of considering initial level of risk. BMJ 1993; 306: 1367-73
16. Committee of Principal Investigators. WHO Cooperative Trial on primary prevention of ischemic heart disease using clofibrate to lower serum cholesterol: mortality follow up. Lancet 1980; II: 379-85
17. Lipid Research Clinics Program. The Lipid Research Clinics Coronary Primary Prevention Trial results: I. Reduction in incidence of coronary heart disease. JAMA 1984; 251: 351-64
18. The Coronary Drug Project Research Group. Clofibrate and niacin in coronary heart disease. JAMA 1975; 231: 360-81
19. Frick MH, Elo MO, Haapa K, et al. Helsinki heart study: primary prevention trial with gemfibrozil in middle-aged men with dyslipidemia. Safety of treatment, changes in risk factors and incidence of coronary heart disease. N Engl J Med 1987; 317: 1237-45
20. Grundy SM. Statin trials and goals of cholesterol-lowering therapy. Circulation 1998; 97: 1436-9
21. West of Scotland Coronary Prevention Study Group. Influence of pravastatin and plasma lipids on clinical events in the West of Scotland Coronary Prevention Study (WOSCOPS). Circulation 1998; 97: 1440-5
22. Pederson TR, Olsson AG, Faergeman O, et al. Lipoprotein changes and reduction in the incidence of major coronary heart disease events in the Scandinavian Simvastatin Study (45). Circulation 1998; 97: 1453-60
23. Post Coronary Artery Bypass Graft Trial Investigators. The effect of aggressive lowering of low-density lipoprotein cholesterol levels and low-dose anticoagulation of obstructive changes in saphenous-vein coronary-artery bypass grafts. N Engl J Med 1997; 336: 153-62
24. Campeau L, Hunninghake DB, Kratterud GŁ, et al. Aggressive cholesterol lowering delays saphenous vein graft atherosclerosis in women, the elderly, and patients with associated risk factors: NHLBI Post Coronary Artery Bypass Graft Clinical Trial. Circulation 1999; 99: 3241-7
25. Pitt B, Waters D, Brown WV, et al. Aggressive lipid-lowering therapy compared with angioplasty in stable coronary artery disease. N Engl J Med 1999; 341: 70-6
26. Jones PH, Kafonek S, Hunninghake D. Comparative dose efficacy study of atorvastatin versus simvastatin, pravastatin, lovastatin and fluvastatin in patients with hypercholesterolemia. Am J Cardiol 1998; 81: 582-7
27. Stein EA, Davidson MH, Dobs HS, et al. Efficacy and safety of simvastatin 80 mg/day in hypercholesterolaemic patients. Am J Cardiol 1998; 82: 311-6
28. Stein E. Cerivastatin in primary hyperlipidemia: a multicenter analysis of efficacy and safety. Am J Cardiol 1998; 82: 40J-6
29. American Diabetes Association. Management of dyslipidemia in adults with diabetes. Diabetes Care 1999; Suppl. I: 56S-9
30. Rubins HB, Robins SJ, Collins D, et al. Gemfibrozil for the secondary prevention of coronary heart disease in men with low levels of high-density lipoprotein cholesterol. N Engl J Med 1999; 341: 410-8

Correspondence: Dr *Peter H. Jones*, Section of Atherosclerosis and Lipid Research, Baylor College of Medicine, 6565 Fannin MS A-601, Houston, TX 77030, USA.
E-mail: jones@bcm.tmc.edu

Pharmacoeconomics of Lipid-Lowering Agents for Primary and Secondary Prevention of Coronary Heart Disease

Joel W. Hay,[1] *Winnie M. Yu*[2] and *Talat Ashraf*[3]

1 Department of Pharmaceutical Economics and Policy, University of Southern California, Los Angeles, California, USA
2 Department of Pharmacy and Therapeutics, University of Pittsburgh, Pittsburgh, Pennsylvania, USA
3 Pharmacoeconomics PPD Inc., Raleigh, North Carolina, USA

Coronary heart disease (CHD) is the leading cause of death in the US, claiming the lives of more than 480 000 Americans in 1995.[1-4] Cardiovascular disease is the leading source of healthcare expenditure in the US and most other industrialised countries. It accounted for $US274 billion in US medical spending and lost output in 1998. Approximately 13.9 million adults have a history of myocardial infarctions or angina pectoris or both.[4] The 5-year cost of CHD has been estimated at $US50 000 per case.[5] Owing to the scarcity of health resources, the escalating cost of healthcare and the high prevalence of CHD, development of cost-effective prevention programmes to reduce the mortality as well as the financial burden of CHD are major national and international priorities.

Hypercholesterolaemia has been identified as an independent modifiable cardiovascular risk factor in several large-scale epidemiological studies and clinical trials. Total serum cholesterol levels exceeding 5.2 mmol/L (200 mg/dl) [mg/dl = mmol/L ÷ 0.02586] were associated with increased risk for initial and subsequent cardiac events such as myocardial infarction (MI), angina pectoris and coronary deaths in the Framingham Heart Study (FHS). The effect of elevated serum cholesterol level is continuous and graded and is multiplicative with other cardiovascular risk factors such as hypertension, cigarette smoking and diabetes mellitus.[6-9]

Cholesterol lowering has been shown to reduce both fatal and nonfatal coronary events in patients with or without CHD.[10-12] It has been proposed that every 1% reduction in total cholesterol level will reduce CHD by 2%.[13,14] Cholesterol lowering by pharmacological or surgical means also prevents atherosclerotic plaque progression, and can even induce regression of atherosclerosis.[15-17] However, until recently, aggressive lipid-lowering therapy remained controversial in the US and elsewhere.

Recently, several large-scale placebo-controlled trials have revisited the relationship between cholesterol reduction and mortality (table I).[19-26] These studies demonstrated significant reductions in coronary events and improvements in survival with the 3-hydroxy-3-methylglutaryl coenzyme A (HMG-CoA) reductase inhibitors, simvastatin and pravastatin.

Table I. Recent primary and secondary prevention studies of hypercholesterolaemia

Clinical trial	Drug/daily dose	Study duration (y)	No. of patients	Sex (ratio: M/F)	Mean age (y)	LDL range (mmol/L)^{a}	Other CHD risk factors^{b} (% of patients)	Major statistically significant results^{c} (% of patients)	Reference
Primary prevention									
LRC-CPPT	Cholestyramine 16 g/day	7.4	3806	1.0/0.0	47.8	5.6 (mean)	Current smoker: 38	LDL: –12 CHD death and/or nonfatal MI: –19 Angina: –20 CABG: –21 Peripheral vascular disease: –15	Lipid Research Clinics Program[13,14]
Helsinki Heart Study	Gemfibrozil 600 mg/day	5.0	4081	1.0/0.0	47.4	5.0 (mean)	Hypertension: 14.5 Current smoker: 36.5	LDL: –8.3 CHD: –64 Nonfatal MI: –37	Frick et al.[18]
WOSCOPS	Pravastatin 40 mg/day	4.9	6595	1.0/0.0	55.0	4.0-6.6	Current smoker: 44	LDL: –26 Nonfatal MI: –31 Cardiac deaths: –32 All-cause mortality: –22 ($p = 0.051$)	Shepherd et al.[19]
AFCAPS/TexCAPS	Lovastatin 20-40 mg/day	5.6	6605	0.85/0.15	58.0	3.4-4.9 (mean 3.9)	Current smoker: 12 Hypertension: 22 Diabetes: 2 HDL <0.91 mmol/L:^{b} 35 Family Hx premature CHD: 16	LDL: –25 1st major coronary event: –36 Unstable angina: –34 Fatal/nonfatal MI: –35 Coronary events: –26 PTCA/CABG: –33	Downs et al.[20]
Secondary prevention									
CDP	Niacin 3 g/day	15.0	8341	1.0/0.0	52.4	6.5 (mean serum cholesterol)	Current smoker: 36.6 Hypertension: 37.4	Total cholesterol: –10.1 All-cause mortality: –11	Canner et al.[10]
4S	Simvastatin 20-40 mg/day	5.4	4444	0.8/0.2	M: 58; F: 60	3.9-6.5^{d}	Current smoker: 27 Hypertension: 26	LDL: –35 Coronary revascularisation: –37 Major coronary events: –29.6 Coronary deaths: –42 All cause mortality: –30	4S Group[21]
PLAC-I and PLAC-II	Pravastatin 40 mg/day	I: 2.4; II: 3	I: 408; II: 151	1.0/0.0	I: 60; II: 57	I: 3.4-5.0; II: 4.2-4.5	Family Hx CHD: 51-71 Hypertension: 25-47 Current smoker: 12-19	Nonfatal MI: –55	Pitt et al.[22], Crouse et al.[23]
CARE	Pravastatin 40 mg/day	5.0	4159	0.86/0.14	59.0	3.0-4.5	Hypertension: 42 Diabetes mellitus: 14 Current smoker: 21	LDL: –32 Coronary revascularisation: –23 Nonfatal MI: –23 Fatal MI: –37 Stroke: –31	Sacks et al.[24]

LIPID	Pravastatin 40 mg/day	>5.0	9014	0.83/0.17	62.0	2.2-5.2	Hypertension: 42 Diabetes mellitus: 9 Current smoker: 10	LDL: −25 Total mortality: −23 Coronary mortality: −24 CABG: −24 Fatal/nonfatal MI: −29 Cardiovascular mortality: −24 Stroke: −20	Tonkin et al.[25]

a For LDL, HDL and total cholesterol levels, mmol/L × 38.7 = mg/dl.
b Only risk factors that occurred in >10% of study population were tabulated.
c Percentage reduction as compared with placebo.
d LDL range is projected to the US population from the 4S total cholesterol study entry criteria and mean study LDL cholesterol levels.

AFCAPS/TexCAPS = Air Force/Texas Coronary Atherosclerosis Prevention Study; **CABG** = coronary artery bypass graft; **CARE** = Cholesterol and Recurrent Events trial; **CDP** = Coronary Drug Project; **CHD** = coronary heart disease; **F** = female; **Hx** = history of; **LDL** = low density lipoprotein cholesterol; **LRC-CPPT** = Lipid Research Clinics Coronary Primary Prevention Trial; **LIPID** = Long-Term Intervention with Pravastatin in Ischaemic Disease study; **M** = male; **MI** = myocardial infarction; **PLAC-I** = Pravastatin Limitation of Atherosclerosis in the Coronary Arteries study; **PLAC-II** = Pravastatin, Lipids, and Atherosclerosis in the Carotid Arteries study; **PTCA** = percutaneous transluminal coronary angioplasty; **WOSCOPS** = West of Scotland Coronary Prevention Study; **4S** = Scandinavian Simvastatin Survival Study.

Drugs of this class (also known as statins) have also been shown in long term intervention and angiographic studies to have excellent efficacy and safety profiles. In particular, the West of Scotland Coronary Prevention Study (WOSCOPS) was a landmark study, in which primary prevention of CHD with pravastatin 40 mg/day significantly reduced the incidence of fatal and nonfatal coronary events in individuals with moderate to severe hypercholesterolaemia. A simple χ^2 analysis of all cause mortality by intention-to-treat showed a 22% reduction in deaths ($p = 0.051$), but the prespecified proportional hazards risk reduction (adjusting for other patient characteristics) was calculated to be 24% ($p = 0.03$).[19]

The Air Force/Texas Coronary Atherosclerosis Prevention Study (AFCAPS/TexCAPS)[20] evaluated the benefits of primary prevention with lovastatin in patients with a mean LDL cholesterol level of 3.9 mmol/L (150 mg/dl). The lovastatin dosage was titrated from 20 mg/day up to 40 mg/day to achieve an LDL cholesterol level goal of ≤2.8 mmol/L (≤110 mg/dl). Preliminary (≥5 years') follow-up showed a 36% reduction in first major acute coronary event ($p < 0.001$) [table I]. Cardiovascular and total mortality were not significantly reduced, probably because of the relatively low risk of mortality in the study population and the lack of statistical power in the study design. The cardiovascular disease event reduction results were consistent for men, women, elderly patients, those with diabetes, smokers and hypertensive patients.

Several secondary prevention trials also support aggressive statin treatment in patients with a history of MI. The Scandinavian Simvastatin Survival Study (4S)[21] was the first study to demonstrate the survival benefit of secondary prevention of CHD. In individuals with moderate to severe hypercholesterolaemia, simvastatin 20 to 40 mg/day significantly reduced major coronary events and total mortality by 35 and 30%, respectively.

The Pravastatin Limitation of Atherosclerosis in the Coronary Arteries (PLAC-I) study[22] and the Pravastatin, Lipids and Atherosclerosis in the Carotid Arteries (PLAC-II) study[23] angiographically examined the effect of pravastatin on the progression of early carotid and coronary atherosclerosis. Pooled analysis of the outcomes of patients in both studies revealed statistically significant reductions in both the incidence of nonfatal MI and in the progression of atherosclerosis (table I).[26] Combining these trials with 2 other angiographic studies in a prespecified meta-analysis, Byington et al.[26] reported that pravastatin significantly reduced fatal and nonfatal MIs and stroke by 62% ($p = 0.0001$).

The Cholesterol and Recurrent Events (CARE) trial,[24] a landmark secondary prevention trial, further demonstrated the clinical benefits of pravastatin in secondary prevention for individuals with normocholesterolemia. The average baseline lipid levels for the CARE population were reflective of a typical North American CHD patient: average total cholesterol level, 5.4 mmol/L (209 mg/dl); LDL cholesterol level, 3.6 mmol/L (139 mg/dl); and high-density lipoprotein (HDL) cholesterol level, 1 mmol/L (39 mg/dl). Overall, statistically significant reductions in nonfatal MI (24%) and fatal MI (37%) were observed in individuals with baseline LDL cholesterol levels as low as 3.0 mmol/L (115 mg/dl). The incidence of stroke was reduced by 31% when compared with placebo ($p = 0.03$). Pravastatin was also proved to be highly beneficial in women and in elderly (≥65 years of age) patients in this trial.[24]

Preliminary results of the Long-Term Intervention with Pravastatin in Ischaemic Disease (LIPID) Study were presented at the 1997 American Heart Association meetings.[25] This Australia/New Zealand study included patients with pre-existing CHD and with baseline LDL cholesterol levels from >2.2 mmol/L (85 mg/dl) to <5.2 mmol/L (<201 mg/dl). As in the CARE and WOSCOPS trials, treated patients were given pravastatin 40 mg/day, while both placebo and treatment patients received dietary and CHD risk factor counselling. The initial findings are presented in table I. A reduction of CHD events in the first 6 to 8 months following therapy initiation was also reported. CHD event reduction results were significant for all study subgroups, including men, women, smokers and nonsmokers, elderly patients and those with hypertension or diabetes.[25]

Despite the demonstrated clinical benefits of statin therapy in both primary and secondary prevention, not all eligible patients receive cholesterol-lowering therapy. In deciding which patients to treat, healthcare policy-makers must weigh the clinical benefits against the economic costs of such treatment. Economic evaluations of the costs and benefits of these agents in patients with different CHD risk factors are essential to guide physicians and health policy-makers in decisions regarding use of scarce healthcare resources. The availability of long-term clinical outcome and mortality data with antihyperlipidemic agents will permit more accurate and comprehensive assessment of potential cost effectiveness and the financial impact of primary and secondary prevention programmes.

Several classes of antihyperlipidemic agents are currently available. These include bile acid-binding resins, fibrates, nicotinic acid and statins. These agents differ in their mechanisms of action, potency in cholesterol lowering, adverse effect profiles, clinical trial outcomes evidence and prices. While clinical trials of antihyperlipidemic agents are suggestive of similar cholesterol reduction benefits across classes of therapies, the possibility of additional and/or separate mechanisms of action for each pharmacological agent weakens generalisations regarding a constant relationship between lipid effects and CHD event reduction.

According to the current US treatment guidelines established by the Adult Treatment Panel of the National Cholesterol Education Program (NCEP) published in 1993,[27] bile acid sequestrants are recommended as first-line agents for primary prevention of CHD in individuals with elevated LDL cholesterol levels and normal triglycerides and in younger adults in whom only moderate reduction in LDL cholesterol levels are necessary. Statins, owing to their high medication costs, are currently reserved for individuals with evident CHD, very high cholesterol levels and multiple CHD risk factors, but the strongly favourable statin outcomes evidence is changing clinical preferences in favour of first-line statin therapy.

For individuals with elevation of both LDL cholesterol and triglycerides levels, nicotinic acid (niacin) is recommended as the drug of first choice.[27] Agents in other classes, particularly the fibrates gemfibrozil and fenofibrate, are reserved for those who have failed niacin therapy.[27] These recommendations were based mainly on medication costs and the limited clinical evidence available at that time.

With the recent availability of new clinical evidence on primary and secondary prevention of CHD, revision of these treatment guidelines is necessary to update the outcomes and cost-effectiveness considerations of these important recommendations. This paper will review published studies and compare the cost effectiveness of different antihyperlipidemic agents. The analytical methods commonly used to analyse the economic benefits of healthcare interventions will also be discussed. All cost-effectiveness ratios within the text were adjusted to 1996 US dollars unless indicated otherwise.

1. Economic Analysis

Four major analytical techniques are commonly used for pharmacoeconomic assessment of healthcare interventions: cost-minimisation analysis, cost-effectiveness analysis, cost-utility analysis and cost-benefit analysis.[28] In the economic evaluation of cardiovascular disease interventions, a specific form of cost-effectiveness analysis – cost per year of life saved (YLS) – is most commonly used. The numerator of this ratio consists of the net incremental cost of the new therapy relative to appropriate current treatment. It includes the cost of medication, treatment initiation, monitoring and managing drug adverse effects minus the cost of medical disease treatment costs avoided because of treatment. The denominator of this ratio is the incremental change in survival resulting from using the new therapy relative to appropriate current treatment.

It may be argued that quality-adjusted life-years gained is the most appropriate method of evaluation in pharmacoeconomic studies.[29] However, few economic models of lipid-lowering strategies have used quality-of-life (QOL) estimates, as accurate and valid measures of these health status variations are generally not available.[30,31] Nevertheless, the QOL differences for alternative lipid-lowering treatments are relatively small in comparison to the survival differences. Generally speaking, a lipid-lowering intervention that has an incremental CHD survival gain of X will produce a total gain of (120 to 130%)X if the QOL changes are included.[32] Particularly for comparisons between statins and surgical or other CHD interventions, ignoring QOL changes increases the cost-effectiveness ratio of the medication, since the QOL impacts of daily use of statins are negligible and the QOL gains from avoiding nonfatal cardiovascular diseases are substantial. Similarly, the QOL impacts of many cardiovascular surgeries and invasive diagnostic procedures can also be substantial. Therefore, adjusting for QOL gains with statin therapy improves (reduces) the cost-effectiveness ratio significantly.[33]

2. Primary Prevention of CHD

According to the current national treatment guidelines established by the Adult Treatment Panel of the NCEP,[27] dietary therapy is recommended as the initial mode of treatment of hypercholesterolaemia. For those who have failed dietary intervention, primary prevention therapies are recommended in individuals with: (i) LDL cholesterol levels >4.9 mmol/L (>190 mg/dl) and fewer than two cardiovascular risk factors; or (ii) LDL cholesterol levels >4.1 mmol/L (>160 mg/dl) and at least 2 cardiovascular risk factors. Following these treatment guidelines, at least 8 million adults are candidates for primary prevention intervention, based on an estimate in 1990.[34]

Owing to the high cost of treatment and the large number of individuals who may benefit from such an intervention, the cost effectiveness of primary prevention programmes has been an area of intense research in the past few years. Of therapies that have been available for a substantial amount of time, the cost effectiveness of bile acid-binding resins and lovastatin have been the most extensively studied.

These pharmacoeconomic analyses have usually projected the hypothetical benefits of cholesterol lowering on CHD risk reduction using multivariate logistic risk equations estimated from the Framingham study cohort.[6,7] The necessary assumption in these analyses is that the relationship between level of relative CHD risk and total serum cholesterol and lipid subfraction levels in an epidemiological study across different individuals can predict the CHD risk reduction achievable in individual patients when medication is used to lower their cholesterol levels. Although predictions from the Framingham study appear to be consistent with other epidemiological studies, prospective outcome data (e.g. the WOSCOPS study) provide a more accurate basis for comprehensive assessment of the CHD risk reduction and cost effectiveness of lipid-lowering interventions such as pravastatin for primary prevention in individuals with hypercholesterolaemia.

Comparative cost-effectiveness estimates reported in the literature for lipid-lowering agents for primary prevention are summarised in tables II and III. In general, any lipid-lowering medication that has a cost-effectiveness ratio ≤$US50 000/year of life saved (YLS) is considered to be acceptably cost effective since the cost-effectiveness ratio is comparable with other well accepted interventions such as chronic haemodialysis, breast cancer screening or coronary artery bypass graft surgery.[48-51]

2.1 Bile Acid-Binding Resins

Two bile acid-binding resins, cholestyramine and colestipol, are currently available in the US. The drugs have similar mechanisms of action and have similar adverse effects. The cost effectiveness of cholestyramine has been more extensively studied than colestipol because of the established clinical efficacy of cholestyramine for primary prevention in reducing the risk of CHD shown in the Lipid Research Clinics Coronary Primary Prevention Trial (LRC-CPPT) trial.[13,14]

2.1.1 Cholestyramine

Weinstein and Stason[36] estimated the cost effectiveness of cholestyramine for primary prevention in men aged between 45 and 50 years and hypercholesterolaemia with serum cholesterol levels >6.9 mmol/L (>265 mg/dl). Assuming full compliance to drug treatment, 24% reduction in CHD mortality and annual therapy cost of $US2000, cholestyramine therapy

Table II. Comparative cost effectiveness of antihyperlipidemic agents for primary prevention of coronary heart disease (CHD)

Drug	Daily dose (g)	Study population charactistics				Cost-effectiveness ratio ($US/YLS) [year]	Cost-effectiveness ratio ($US/YLS, 1996 values)	Reference
		gender	age (y)	TC or LDL (mmol/L)[a]	other CHD risk factors			
Soluble fibre								
Oat bran	90	M	48	> 6.9	Current smoker: 38%	9200 [1985]	17 800	Kinosian & Eisenberg[35]
Bile acid binding resins								
Cholestyramine	24	M	45-59	> 6.9	None	126 000 [1984]	263 300	Weinstein & Stason[36]
	16.8	M	48	7.2	Current smoker: 38%	117 400 [1985]	227 800	Kinosian & Eisenberg[35]
	24	NS	NS	> 6.5	None	347/1% LDL reduction [1989]	534/1% LDL reduction	Schulman et al.[37]
	16[b]	M	35-74	6.9	None	102 100-777 600 [1985]	198 000-1 508 500	Oster & Epstein[38]
	12[c]	M	35-60	8.0	None	NLG208 000-NLG483 000[d] [1988]	171 600-398 500	Martens et al.[39], Martens & Rutten[40]
Colestipol	22	M	48	7.2	Current smoker: 38%	63 500 [1985]	123 200	Kinosian & Eisenberg[35]
Fibrates								
Gemfibrozil	1.2	NS	NS	> 6.5	None	330/1% LDL reduction [1989]	508/1% LDL reduction	Schulman et al.[37]
	1.2	M	40	> 6.9	1 CHD risk factor	108 826 [1987]	189 400	Kelley[41]
Nicotinic acid								
Niacin	3	NS	NS	> 6.5	None	139/1% LDL reduction [1989]	214/1% LDL reduction	Schulman et al.[37]
	3	M	40	> 6.5	1 CHD risk factor	8 500 [1987]	14 900	Kelley[41]

a For TC, mmol/L × 38.7 = mg/dl.
b 378g bulk dosage form.
c Unit dose of 4 g/package.
d NLG2 = $US1.
M = male; **NS** = not stated; **LDL** = low density lipoprotein; **NLG** = Dutch guiders; **TC** = total cholesterol; **YLS** = year of life saved.

Table III. Comparative cost effectiveness of HMG-CoA reductase inhibitors for primary prevention of coronary heart disease (CHD)

Statin	Daily dose (mg)	Study population characteristics: gender	age (y)	TC, LDL or HDL (mmol/L)[a]	other CHD risk factors	Cost-effectiveness ratio ($US/YLS, except where specified) [year]	Cost-effectiveness ratio ($US/YLS, 1996 values)	Reference
Lovastatin	20	NS	NS	TC: >6.5	None	177/1% LDL reduction [1989]	273/1% LDL reduction	Schulman et al.[37]
	20	M	45-74	TC: >7.8	≥1[b]	13 000-38 000 [1989]	20 200-58 500	Goldman et al.[42]
	20	M	45-74	TC: 6.5-7.7	≥2[b]	27 000-37 000 [1989]	41 600-57 000	Goldman et al.[42]
	20	F	55-74	TC: >7.8	≥2[b]	34 000-39 000 [1989]	52 400-60 100	Goldman et al.[42]
	20	M	35-55	TC: 5.4-9.8	SBP: 180mm Hg	6 000-38 000 [1989]	9 200-58 500	Hay et al.[33]
	20	F	35-55	TC: 5.4-9.8	SBP: 180mm Hg	19 000-89 000 [1989]	29 300-137 100	Hay et al.[33]
	20	M	30-70	TC: 6.6-7.2	DBP: 100mm Hg	$Can20 882-$Can50 079[c] [1992]	18 900-45 300	Hamilton et al.[43]
	20	F	30-70	TC: 6.3-8.0	DBP: 100mm Hg	$Can36 627-$Can105 708[c] [1992]	33 100-95 500	Hamilton et al.[43]
	20	M	45	LDL: 4.5	Current smoker	$Can53 000[c] [1993]	44 800	Martens & Guibert[44]
Fluvastatin	40	M	45	LDL: 4.5	Current smoker	$Can38 800[c] [1993]	32 800	Martens & Guibert[44]
	40	M	45	LDL: 3.5-5.5	Current smoker	$Can21 600-$Can27 800[c] [1993]	18 200-23 500	Martens & Guibert[44]
Pravastatin	40	M	45-64	TC: 7.0 LDL: 4.9 HDL: 1.1	Current smoker: 44% Diabetes: 1% DBP: 84mm Hg	£20 375[d] [1996]	31 700	WOSCOPS Economic Analysis Group[45]
	40	M	45	TC: 7.0 LDL: 4.9 HDL: 1.1	Current smoker: 44% Diabetes: 1% DBP: 84mm Hg	13 600 [1996]	13 600	Hay et al.[46]
	40	M	49	TC: 6.8	Current smoker: 48% DBP: 84mm Hg	61 000 [1991]	77 900	Johannesson et al.[47]
Simvastatin	20	M	35-60	TC: 8.0	None	NLG46 000-NLG98 000[e] [1988]	23 000–49 000	Martens et al.,[39] Martens & Rutten[40]
	10	M	45	LDL: 4.5	Current smoker	$Can48 300 [1993]	40 800	Martens & Guibert[44]

a For LDL, HDL and TC, mmol/L × 38.7 = mg/dl.
b CHD risk factors such as hypertension, smoking and obesity.
c $Can1.35 = $US1.
d £0.62 = $US1.
e NLG2 = $US1.

CHD = coronary heart disease; **DBP** = diastolic blood pressure; **F** = female; **HDL** = high density lipoprotein; **LDL** = low density lipoprotein; **M** = male; **NLG** = Dutch guilders; **NS** = not stated; **SBP** = systolic blood pressure; **TC** = total cholesterol; **YLS** = year of life saved; **$Can** = Canadian dollars.

24 g/day was found to be highly cost ineffective, with base case cost per YLS of $US263 400 (adjusted to 1996 values). The cost effectiveness of cholestyramine in other age groups and populations, with other CHD risk factors were not examined in the study. The costs of therapy monitoring and the indirect benefits such as cost savings because of gain in productivity from avoided disease were not included in the analysis. Study perspective was not specified by the authors.

In another analysis, Oster and Epstein[38] examined the cost effectiveness of cholestyramine (16 g/day) for primary prevention of CHD from a societal perspective. The effects of age, duration of treatment and pretreatment cholesterol level on the cost-effectiveness ratio were also evaluated. Framingham multivariate logistic risk equations were used to estimate CHD risk as a function of total serum cholesterol level and other CHD risk factors. Treatment benefits were assumed to begin 2 years after initiation of therapy. Both direct and indirect resource costs were included with future costs and benefits discounted at an annual rate of 5%. Cost effectiveness of cholestyramine ranged from $US69 000 to over $US1 million per YLS, depending on the CHD risk profile of the study patient. In general, cholestyramine was not cost effective except in patients aged 35 to 44 years old with pretreatment cholesterol levels ≥7.5 mmol/L (≥290 mg/dl) and at least 3 coronary risk factors such as smoking, hypertension and diabetes mellitus. Life-long treatment was not as cost effective as treatment of limited-term and cost effectiveness generally peaked at 5 to 10 years after initiation of therapy. Cost effectiveness improved (cost-effectiveness ratio decreased) with decreasing age at initiation of therapy, increasing pretreatment cholesterol level, increasing number of CHD risk factors and decreasing daily dosages.

Similar findings were obtained in the cost-effectiveness analysis by Kinosian and Eisenberg.[35] Primary prevention using cholestyramine was generally not cost effective, with cost-effectiveness ratios greater than $US50 000/YLS in most cases. Cost effectiveness improves in younger patients and in high risk patients who have multiple CHD risk factors.

2.1.2 Colestipol

Colestipol has been shown to significantly reduce CHD deaths in high risk men who have a serum cholesterol level of 7.8 mmol/L (302 mg/dl), although a mortality difference was not observed in women treated with colestipol.[52] Using efficacy data for primary prevention with cholestyramine in the LRC-CPTT trial,[13,14] and assuming the efficacy of colestipol to be equivalent to that of cholestyramine (an unproven assumption), Kinosian and Eisenberg[35] performed an economic simulation of a 7-years' intervention with colestipol. Both direct and indirect costs of nonfatal events were included in the analysis and future costs and benefits were discounted at 5% annually. In 48-year-old men with total serum cholesterol levels ≥6.9 mmol/L (≥265 mg/dl) and no other CHD risk factor except for a smoking prevalence of 38%, the cost effectiveness of colestipol (22 g/day, bulk drug) was found to be similar to that of cholestyramine (16.8 g/day, bulk drug), with a cost-effectiveness ratio of $US123 700/YLS. Using the drug in packet form rather than in bulk form significantly increased the cost-effectiveness ratio since the unit dose form was more expensive than the bulk form. Oat bran 90 g/day was projected to be more cost effective than colestipol and cholestyramine, with a cost-effectiveness ratio of 75% lower than that of either agent in patients with similar CHD risks.[35] Whether supplementation of dietary fibre such as oat bran to low cholesterol diet offers an attractive strategy for dietary modification in high risk patients depends on dietary compliance and the degree of cholesterol lowering needed.[53]

2.2 Fibric Acid Derivatives

Gemfibrozil and clofibrate are two fibric acid derivatives that have been approved for use in the US. Fenofibrate is another fibric acid derivative that is marketed in many other countries and has recently been approved in the US. Gemfibrozil is more commonly used than clofibrate because of its well established clinical efficacy and favourable adverse effect profile. It decreases LDL cholesterol levels, increases HDL cholesterol levels and has been shown to significantly reduce cardiac events when used for primary prevention of CHD in middle-aged men with hypercholesterolaemia.[18] However, few economic analyses have been performed to examine its potential cost effectiveness.

Schulman et al.[37] compared the cost effectiveness of gemfibrozil 1.2 g/day to other anti-hyperlipidemic agents from a societal perspective. Cost effectiveness was computed as cost of therapy per percentage reduction in LDL cholesterol level. Costs of therapy included cost of drug treatment, monitoring and treating possible adverse effects; however, averted resource costs due to prevented outcomes and indirect benefits such as gain in wages and productivity were not considered in the calculation. Costs were discounted to present value at a rate of 5%.

Comparing the cost per percentage reduction in LDL cholesterol level, gemfibrozil and cholestyramine appeared to be similar at approximately $US460 for every percentage point reduction in LDL. The costs per percentage reduction in LDL ratio with niacin 3 g/day and lovastatin 20 mg/day were approximately half those of gemfibrozil because of their higher potencies in LDL reduction and lower costs of therapy. Since these lipid-lowering agents may differ in their efficacies and mechanisms of action, long term therapeutic outcomes achieved by these agents may differ. Therefore, comparing cost-effectiveness ratios that are expressed in terms of cost per percentage reduction in LDL cholesterol level may not allow accurate assessment of the relative cost effectiveness of these agents.

Kelley evaluated the cost effectiveness of gemfibrozil from a societal perspective.[41] Using an assumption that each incident of symptomatic CHD cost $US41 000 in direct medical expenses and indirect loss of earnings, and every 1% reduction in total cholesterol level resulted in 0.93 months increase in life expectancy, gemfibrozil 1.2 g/day was not found to be cost effective in 40-year-old-men with total cholesterol levels >6.9 mmol/L (>265 mg/dl) [$US189 400/YLS adjusted to 1996 values]. However, if the benefit of increasing HDL cholesterol levels was incorporated in the analysis, the projected cost-effectiveness ratio would be reduced by 50% or more. Moreover, gemfibrozil is now available in a much cheaper generic formulation. Taking these factors into consideration, we calculated that the projected cost per YLS with gemfibrozil would be substantially less than $US40 000.

In another study by Syam and Fifer,[54] the potential economic benefits of gemfibrozil for primary prevention of CHD were analysed using a cost-benefit approach. The 5-year probability of a CHD event, defined as acute MI or sudden death, for an individual aged 45 to 55 years with a total cholesterol level of 7.0 mmol/L (270 mg/dl) was estimated based on data from the Helsinki Heart Study. Taking into account the benefit of gemfibrozil on HDL cholesterol levels, the net cost of gemfibrozil therapy for an averted CHD event such as acute MI and sudden death ranged from $US200 to $US500 per year, with the highest cost in the lowest risk group. The economic benefits of gemfibrozil therapy might have been understated in the study since additional savings due to other averted cardiac events such as angina pectoris and recurrent ischaemic events were not considered in the analysis.

Extending these findings to a public health intervention programme such as the Medi-Cal programme and assuming gemfibrozil treatment in 13 000 individuals with moderate to high risk for CHD, total net programme savings attributed to gemfibrozil therapy were projected to be greater than $US5 million per year (1990 values). Cost-effectiveness (in terms of dollars per YLS) and cost-benefit ratios were not calculated in the study.

No clinical trials have been conducted to determine the effects of fenofibrate on morbidity and mortality, and there is little pharmacoeconomic literature on this medication, despite its favourable impact on serum triglycerides and HDL cholesterol levels. A Canadian study projected fenofibrate to be relatively cost effective, but this analysis was based on epidemiological models projecting disease reduction benefits from changes in surrogate lipid markers.[55]

2.3 Nicotinic Acid

Nicotinic acid (i.e. niacin) is currently recommended by the Adult Treatment Panel of the NCEP as the first-line treatment for individuals with elevated LDL cholesterol and triglyceride levels.[27] Niacin favourably affects lipids and lipoproteins by decreasing LDL cholesterol and triglyceride levels and increasing HDL cholesterol levels. The cost effectiveness of niacin has not been extensively evaluated since information regarding its efficacy in reducing coronary events in primary prevention is lacking, and the data for secondary prevention are also limited.

Schulman et al.[37] expressed cost-effectiveness in terms of cost of societal resource consumption per percentage reduction in LDL cholesterol level. Direct medical costs such as medication costs, physician visit costs and laboratory costs and costs of treating possible adverse effects were considered. When compared with other agents such as cholestyramine, lovastatin or gemfibrozil, niacin appeared to be the most cost effective for reducing LDL cholesterol levels, with a cost-effectiveness ratio of $US139 per percentage reduction in LDL levels in individuals with total cholesterol levels >6.5 mmol/L (>250 mg/dl) [1989 values]. However, this study did not take into account intangible costs, such as unpleasantness of the medication, lack of tolerability and noncompliance. The study also assumed that the impact of niacin on CHD event reduction was fully characterised by Framingham equations relating CHD risk changes to changes in lipid values.

Kelley[41] examined the cost effectiveness of niacin in 40-year-old men with total cholesterol levels >6.9 mmol/L (>265 mg/dl) and one CHD risk factor from the perspective of society. Net cost was defined as cost of medications, monitoring and adverse effect treatment minus cost of diseases avoided and extra income earned from the averted diseases. Assuming niacin 3 g/day reduced LDL cholesterol levels by 20% and a treatment duration of 30 years, the cost-effectiveness ratio of niacin was found to be $US14 900/YLS (adjusted to 1996 values), with costs and benefits discounted at 5% *per annum*. This was based on an epidemiological projection of disease reduction benefits since no primary prevention study with niacin has ever been conducted.

2.4 Statins

In the past 10 years, 6 statins (lovastatin, pravastatin, simvastatin, fluvastatin, atorvastatin and cerivastatin) have been approved as adjuncts to diet for treatment of type IIa and IIb hypercholesterolaemia.[56,57] These agents are the most potent LDL cholesterol-lowering drugs available, and are also the best tolerated of the available lipid-lowering medications. Despite the similarities of these agents in their major mechanisms of action on circulating lipids, they differ in potency, efficacy and price.

The statins may also differ in other important mechanisms of action affecting coronary plaque development that might substantially impact the risk of CHD.[58] Potential areas of difference include smooth muscle cell inhibition, antithrombotic effects, inflammatory and immune system activation, plaque collagen matrix stabilisation, lipid oxidation, lipid subfraction modification and possibly other factors. How these mechanisms differ among the statins, and how important these additional mechanisms are to clinical outcomes is under active investigation by research cardiologists. Similar investigations are also proceeding for the non-statin cholesterol-lowering agents.

Lovastatin was the first statin available in the US. Clinical evidence on slowing atherosclerosis and prevention of primary CHD has been recently demonstrated for lovastatin.[20] Pravastatin has been shown to improve survival in both primary and secondary prevention of CHD in large scale, randomised placebo-controlled trials, and to reduce risk cardiovascular events in clinical trials encompassing patients reflecting all subgroups recommended for pharmacological treatment under the NCEP guidelines.[19,22-25] Simvastatin has also been demonstrated to improve survival in secondary prevention of CHD among patients with hypercholesterolaemia.[21] Fluvastatin is the least potent statin in terms of LDL cholesterol level reduction, but the least expensive in terms of acquisition cost among all statin agents. Atorvastatin and cerivastatin, the most potent LDL cholesterol-reducing agents, have recently been approved for use in the US and elsewhere. No data on clinical event reduction exist for fluvastatin, cerivastatin or atorvastatin.

With the availability of these statins, each with unique characteristics, healthcare professionals face difficult decisions in treatment of hypercholesterolaemia and heart disease. Trade-offs between cost, potency and evidence of actual outcomes effectiveness need to be considered carefully in making treatment decisions.

2.4.1 Lovastatin

Based on projections of the benefits of lipid-lowering from the FHS, lovastatin appears to be reasonably cost effective compared with other well accepted medical practices. Goldman et al.[42] estimated the potential cost effectiveness of lovastatin from the societal perspective using a computer-simulation Coronary Heart Disease Policy Model. The model used the 30-year follow-up data from the FHS and computed individuals' risk for CHD based on their CHD risk factors, total serum cholesterol levels and CHD status. Only direct costs of coronary disease were taken into account in the analysis. Clinical benefits were assumed to begin 2 years after initiation of lovastatin therapy and future benefits were discounted at an annual rate of 5%. Cost effectiveness of lovastatin at different dosages, in different age groups and in individuals with moderate [total cholesterol levels of 6.5 to 7.7 mmol/L (250 to 299 mg/dl)] and severe [total cholesterol levels ≥7.8 mmol/L (≥300 mg/dl)] hypercholesterolaemia were analysed.

For men with total cholesterol levels ≥7.8 mmol/L (≥300 mg/dl), lovastatin 20 mg/day was cost effective (<$US50 000/YLS) only in (i) individuals aged 45 to 74 years who were hypertensive; and (ii) selected high risk groups aged 35 to 44 years who were hypertensive (diastolic blood pressure ≥105mm Hg), cigarette smokers and obese individuals (≥130% ideal bodyweight). Lovastatin was not cost effective in patients aged 75 to 84 years, with a cost-effectiveness ratio greater than $US92 615/YLS in all risk groups. Similarly, for women with cholesterol levels ≥7.8 mmol/L (≥300 mg/dl), lovastatin 20 mg/day was cost effective only in high risk patients aged 55 to 74 years who smoked and were hypertensive and obese. Increasing the lovastatin dosage from 20 to 40 mg/day increased the cost-effectiveness ratio by at least $US50 000/YLS in all patients. In patients with only moderate hypercholesterolaemia, lovastatin was generally much less cost effective, with a cost-effectiveness ratio of less than $US40 000/YLS only in high risk groups aged 55 to 74 years with at least 2 CHD risk factors.

This analysis did not consider direct costs for noncoronary disease or indirect benefits such as gain in productivity secondary to averted coronary disease. Estimating the risk for CHD based solely on total cholesterol levels may have underestimated the economic benefits of lovastatin therapy since the potential benefits of increased HDL cholesterol level was ignored.

Hay et al.[33] evaluated the costs and benefits of lovastatin for primary prevention of CHD. Cost effectiveness for CHD reduction in individuals with different CHD risk factors and cholesterol levels were estimated from Framingham multivariate logistic risk equations based on projections from serum lipid changes. Net costs were defined as intervention and adverse effect costs minus reduction in medical costs due to averted cardiac events. Future benefits were discounted to present values at an annual rate of 5%. In low risk normotensive individuals aged 35 to 55 years, lovastatin was projected to be cost effective only in men with total serum cholesterol levels ≥6.7 mmol/L (≥260 mg/dl) with cost-effectiveness ratios in the range of $US13 892/YLS to $US44 764/YLS, depending on the smoking status of the individual. Applying the same intervention to high risk individuals aged 35 to 55 years with systolic hypertension (systolic blood pressure = 180mm Hg), cost effectiveness improved dramatically, with favourable cost-effectiveness ratios in patients with total cholesterol levels as low as 5.4 mmol/L (208 mg/dl). Cost effectiveness was relatively insensitive to medical care costs, suggesting that the main benefits of lovastatin were due to gains in life expectancy rather than reduction in medical costs. The estimate did take into account the risk reduction due to increased HDL cholesterol level but it did not consider indirect cost savings due to gain in wages and labour productivity from averted coronary events.

Hamilton et al.[43] evaluated the lifetime cost effectiveness of lovastatin for primary prevention of CHD, taking into account the benefits of both decreasing total cholesterol and increasing HDL cholesterol levels. Benefits of CHD risk factor modification were estimated using the CHD prevention model, a model derived from FHS data. Cost effectiveness was defined as net costs per net gain in life expectancy. Net costs included medication costs, savings due to averted cardiovascular events and additional expenditures due to noncoronary diseases as a result of increased life expectancy. This latter cost (medical costs for treating noncoronary diseases due to increased survival from treatment) is a valid consideration for studies conducted from the healthcare payer perspective (e.g. the government in Canada), but not for studies conducted from a societal perspective since such costs are not part of the societal burden of heart disease.

Assuming lovastatin 20 mg/day reduced total serum cholesterol levels by 17% and increased HDL cholesterol levels by 7%, lovastatin 20 mg/day was most cost effective in high risk men (smokers, diastolic blood pressure of 100mm Hg and total cholesterol level at or above the 90th percentile corresponding to their age and gender) aged 30 to 60 years and women aged 50 to 70 years, with a cost-effectiveness ratio of less than 43 000 Canadian dollars ($Can)/YLS (1993 values) equivalent to approximately $US30 000/YLS (1996 values).[43] In general, the cost-effectiveness ratio was lower in men and in high risk groups. When the beneficial effects on HDL cholesterol levels were taken into account, approximately a 40% reduction in the cost-effectiveness ratio was observed. Indirect benefits due to gains in productivity and direct costs to treat possible adverse effects were not considered in the analysis.

The incremental cost effectiveness of lovastatin 20 mg/day relative to fluvastatin 40 mg/day and other statins for primary prevention of CHD in Canada was evaluated in a study by Martens and Guibert.[44] Instead of estimating the CHD risk based on total cholesterol or total cholesterol and HDL cholesterol levels, this study expressed CHD risk as a function of LDL and HDL cholesterol levels. A mathematical model derived from the Canadian Heart Health Survey and FHS data was used to estimate the lifetime CHD risk. Net costs included both savings incurred secondary to averted cardiac events and the lifetime costs of cholesterol lowering such as drug cost and monitoring costs; however, indirect costs and non-CHD medical costs were not considered. The cost effectiveness of lovastatin 20 mg/day in 45-year-old men who smoked and had pretreatment LDL cholesterol levels of 4.5 mmol/L (175 mg/dl) was $Can53 000/YLS (1993 values), equivalent to approximately $45 000/YLS (1996 values). The incremental cost-effectiveness ratio of lovastatin 20 mg/day relative to fluvastatin 40 mg/day was $Can198 100/YLS (1993 values) or $US146 000/YLS (1996 values). Cost effectiveness of lovastatin in populations with other CHD risk factors was not evaluated. The higher cost-effectiveness ratio observed in this study compared with those from US analyses is probably due to lower healthcare costs and rates of use in Canada.[59] The differences in medication costs and the prevalence of CHD risk factors between Canada and US may also have contributed to the difference in the cost effectiveness observed.

2.4.2 Pravastatin

Despite the well established clinical efficacy of pravastatin in cholesterol lowering, few studies have evaluated the benefits of pravastatin economically. Johannesson et al.[47] used the Framingham risk equations to project the cost effectiveness of pravastatin for primary prevention in the Swedish Cost Effectiveness of Lipid Lowering (CELL) study population. The costs were defined as cost of intervention (e.g. medications, laboratory tests, etc.) minus the cost saved due to reduction in cardiovascular morbidity. Healthcare costs due to increased survival were not included and all costs and life-years were discounted by 5%. In a middle-aged male population who had a serum cholesterol level of 6.8 mmol/L (264 mg/dl), diastolic blood pressure of 83.5mm Hg and in which 48% were smokers, a cholesterol-lowering programme that consisted of usual advice and pravastatin therapy of 2 years in duration was found to be not cost effective, with a cost-effectiveness ratio of $US61 000/YLS (1991 values).

As described above (section 2.4.1), Martens and Guibert[44] compared the cost effectiveness of several statins in Canada. In this study, the cost effectiveness of pravastatin 20 mg/day was $Can56 200/YLS (1993 values), or $US47 500/YLS at 1996 values.

The WOSCOPS Economic Analysis Group performed a cost-effectiveness study of pravastatin using both the clinical trial results and Scottish life expectancy data to determine cost effectiveness in the UK. They found a base case cost-effectiveness ratio of £20 375 per YLS ($US33 060 per YLS using 1997 values; monetary conversion may not directly translate value of resources used) for men aged 45 to 64 years (benefits discounted at 6% annually).[45]

Also using WOSCOPS clinical data, we conservatively estimated the cost effectiveness of pravastatin for primary prevention in the US using the data reported for the clinical trial period and the reported CHD event and mortality reduction rates.[19] Depending on the individual's

CHD risk factor profile, using an 'intent-to-treat' analysis, the pravastatin cost-effectiveness ratio ranged from $US11 000/YLS to $US50 000/YLS (1997 values) over the 5.6 years of clinical trial follow-up.

Economic evaluation of the WOSCOPS study also demonstrates that the on-treatment CHD event risk reduction achieved with pravastatin in primary prevention is about 50% better than the event risk reduction predicted from Framingham equations based on average patient changes in HDL and LDL lipid values alone.[46] This raises the question of whether epidemiological risk reduction models using Framingham equations (or other risk equations) based on surrogate markers such as changes in serum cholesterol levels are valid predictors of actual event risk reduction with any specific medication such as pravastatin.

2.4.3 Simvastatin

Few studies have been published on the cost effectiveness of simvastatin for primary prevention (table III). The cost effectiveness of simvastatin 20 mg/day has been compared with cholestyramine 12 g/day in the context of the Dutch healthcare system using a CHD risk reduction model projected from Framingham multivariate logistic risk functions.[39,40] For middle-aged men with an initial serum cholesterol level of 8.0 mmol/L (310 mg/dl), simvastatin was substantially more cost effective than cholestyramine, with a cost-effectiveness ratio ranging from $US23 000 to $US49 000/YLS depending on the patients' age at initiation of therapy. Medication costs and costs of treating symptomatic CHD were included in the analysis, with all costs and benefits discounted to present value at 5% *per annum*. The cost-effectiveness ratio was sensitive to medication and treatment costs, suggesting that these results may not be applicable to the US population due to the difference in health resource costs between the 2 countries. The high serum cholesterol level of the study patients [8 mmol/L (310 mg/dl)] occurs in less than 5% of the US population, also limiting the usefulness of the study results in the US.

The cost effectiveness of simvastatin 10 mg/day in Canada was estimated and compared with other statins by Martens and Guibert[44] (section 2.4.1). The cost-effectiveness ratio of simvastatin was found to be $Can48 300/YLS (1993 values), or $US40 800/YLS at 1996 values. Simvastatin 10 mg/day was not projected to be as cost effective as fluvastatin 40 mg/day, with an incremental cost-effectiveness ratio of $Can88 200/YLS (1993 values) [$US74 500/YLS at 1996 values] in individuals with the same CHD risk profile. Nevertheless, these results are not based on actual outcomes data, but rather projections from Framingham risk reduction equations.

2.4.4 Fluvastatin

Being the least expensive statin in the US market, fluvastatin has been described as the 'most cost effective' lipid-lowering agent.[60-62] However, these reports should be interpreted with caution since their estimates were based solely on the projected cost to reduce LDL cholesterol levels by 1%, rather than on total costs and outcomes of lipid therapy. In order to fully assess the true pharmacoeconomic effects of a lipid-lowering agent, it is important to consider the long term benefits such as reduction in cardiac events and improvement in overall survival. No clinical evidence of prevention of cardiac events such as MI or angina pectoris exists for fluvastatin; however, large, long term studies have not been conducted. Studies with other agents have shown that reduction in such events can offset drug costs by 100% or more, especially in individuals with high CHD risk.[63,64] Therefore, projecting cost effectiveness based solely on drug costs and lipid effects may understate the cost effectiveness of other agents and overstate the cost effectiveness of fluvastatin.[22,23,26]

In the study described in section 2.4.1, Martens and Guibert[44] evaluated the cost effectiveness of several statins, including fluvastatin, in Canada. The estimated cost-effectiveness ratio for fluvastatin 40 mg/day in the study population ranged from $Can21 600 to $Can63 900/YLS (1993 values) or $US18 200 to $US54 000/YLS (1996 values), depending upon the CHD risk profile.

A more recent retrospective data evaluation also implies that fluvastatin is the most cost effective statin.[65] However, several flaws in this study are apparent. First, LDL cholesterol reduction is used as the only measure of effectiveness, in absence of data on other changes in lipids or true disease outcomes data. Second, although termed a randomised study, this evaluation is in fact a retrospective evaluation of patients who (at the advice of their doctors) chose one of several statin therapies. In addition, patients were excluded from the study if they: (i) discontinued statin therapy in the first 60 days; (ii) began combination therapy (e.g. statin plus bile acid sequestrant); or (iii) died. These exclusions could bias the study conclusions.

Similarly, another study which compares the cost effectiveness of different statins and fibrates[55] is based on comparative lipid-lowering data from a single clinical trial, projected to CHD risk reduction [using methodology similar to that of Shulman et al.[37] (section 2.2)]. The analysis is done within the Canadian healthcare context. The authors conclude that primary CHD prevention in patients with hyperlipidaemia is generally cost effective for statin and fibrate medications, using a cost effectiveness cutpoint of $US50 000/YLS.

2.4.5 Atorvastatin

One paper has been published on the costs of atorvastatin treatment.[66] The analysis compared the direct medical costs for patients randomised to atorvastatin, simvastatin, lovastatin or fluvastatin over a 54-week period in 30 centres. The analysis found that the average total cost of care with atorvastatin (including physician visits, drug costs, laboratory tests and other monitoring costs) was $US1064. This is more than $US400 less than similar costs for the other statins. This cost study is not based on outcomes data, and merely presents the cost of achieving LDL cholesterol reduction goals as specified by the NCEP Adult Treatment Panel. The analysis therefore suffers from many of the same problems associated with the fluvastatin study described earlier.[65] Moreover, patients discontinuing therapy because of lack of response were lost to follow-up.

A recently completed outcomes study, the Atorvastatin Versus Revascularization Treatments (AVERT) trial is quite promising in suggesting that atorvastatin may produce many of the beneficial risk reductions demonstrated by pravastatin, simvastatin and lovastatin, and may also be highly cost effective, at least in patients with symptomatic CHD.[67] Results from the AVERT trial demonstrated that 87% of patients randomised to atorvastatin, who were originally candidates for angioplasty, were instead able to remain on this medical therapy for the duration of the 18-month trial period, without experiencing any cardiovascular events. In addition, patients who received atorvastatin had a 36% reduction in the combined incidence of cardiovascular events, such as nonfatal heart attacks, bypass surgery, revascularisation and worsening angina, as compared with patients receiving angioplasty followed by usual care. Unfortunately, probably because of the small sample size (n = 341) and limited follow-up period (18 months), these CHD end-point results were not statistically significant. There was no difference in the incidence of 'hard end-points' (cardiovascular death, cerebrovascular accident, MI, cardiac arrest), 5 with Lipitor and 6 with usual care. Nevertheless, significant reductions in the number of coronary artery bypass grafts performed and cases with worsening of angina were observed in the atorvastatin treatment arm. This is yet another statin study demonstrating important outcomes benefits, but over a short study period. Other outcomes studies [e.g. Treating to New Targets (TNT) trial and Myocardial Ischemia Reduction with Aggressive Cholesterol Lowering (MIRACL) trial are underway which will provide additional data to refine the estimates of the cost effectiveness of atorvastatin.

2.4.6 Cerivastatin

At the time of writing, long term outcome studies on the efficacy of cerivastatin in CHD events reduction are not available. However, based on current US pricing, it can be projected that cost per percentage change in LDL cholesterol levels will be more favourable with cerivastatin than with the other statins. This begs the question as to whether LDL potency is a valid proxy for genuine CHD event and mortality risk reduction, and whether short term safety and efficacy trials adequately reflect long term drug tolerability and effectiveness.

3. Secondary Prevention

According to the American Heart Association estimate, over 6 million adults currently have evident CHD.[4] Following the current NCEP treatment guidelines for secondary prevention [LDL cholesterol level >3.4 mmol/L (>130 mg/dl) with pre-existing CHD], it was estimated that approximately 4 million adults in the US were candidates for secondary prevention of CHD in 1990.[27,34] Drug treatment of hypercholesterolaemia in patients with overt CHD has remained controversial until recently. The CARE,[24] PLAC-I,[22] PLAC-II,[23] LIPID and 4S[21] studies have proven the clinical efficacy of pravastatin and simvastatin in the context of secondary prevention. With pravastatin, clinical benefits were seen not only in patients with hypercholesterolaemia but also in normocholesterolemic individuals with a baseline LDL cholesterol level averaging 3.6 mmol/L (139 mg/dl). These studies therefore lend support to the use of a more aggressive approach towards cholesterol modification such as initiation of drug treatment in individuals with pre-existing heart disease and baseline LDL cholesterol levels of ≥3.0 mmol/L (≥115 mg/dl).

Although only a few studies have evaluated the cost effectiveness of secondary prevention, the results are highly favourable.

Prior to the availability of the clinical outcome data from 4S, LIPID and CARE, Goldman et al.[42] estimated the hypothetical cost effectiveness of lovastatin in subgroups with mild to moderate [<6.5 mmol/L (<250 mg/dl)] and moderate to severe [>6.5 mmol/L (>250 mg/dl)] hypercholesterolaemia. Framingham risk equations were used to estimate the CHD incidence and all-cause mortality in groups with different age and gender. Only direct medical costs were included in the analysis and costs and benefits were discounted at 5% *per annum*. Assuming secondary prevention programmes using lovastatin reduced CHD risk by the same extent as primary prevention programmes and that every 1% reduction in serum cholesterol level reduced cardiac events by 1.9%, lovastatin 20 mg/day was found to be cost effective in men and women of all ages with moderate to severe elevation of serum cholesterol levels [>6.46 mmol/L (>250 mg/dl)], with cost-effectiveness ratios of less than $US31 000/YLS (1989 values).

Within the same subgroup, lovastatin therapy was found to save lives *and* money in men aged 35 to 54 years. A 40 mg/day dosage was also cost effective in all men but less favourable in women, with incremental cost-effectiveness ratios of $US44 800 to $US75 700/YLS. Although less cost effective than in those with higher serum cholesterol levels, treatment in subgroups with serum cholesterol levels <6.5 mmol/L (<250 mg/dl) was cost effective in men of all ages and in women aged 55 to 84 years, with cost-effectiveness ratios of less than $US61 700/YLS. Treatment in this subgroup using a 40 mg/day dosage was also less cost effective than in the high risk group with serum cholesterol levels >6.5 mmol/L (250 mg/dl). Higher doses such as 80 mg/day were not cost effective in both subgroups, with the incremental cost-effectiveness ratio consistently greater than $US108 000/YLS in all men and women.

Although numerous studies have used Framingham risk equations for CHD risk projection, the applicability of these equations in projecting the CHD risk in populations that have not been studied in clinical trials such as the elderly or women is uncertain.[13,14,68,69]

Published analyses of the 4S, PLAC-I and PLAC-II results suggest that these agents are highly cost effective in most patients, with base-case cost-effectiveness ratios less than $US20 000/YLS for simvastatin and less than $US10 000 for pravastatin.[64,70] There are even cost savings in patients at sufficiently high risk.[71]

In a recent cost-minimisation study that evaluated the benefits of cholesterol lowering from the 4S study data, simvastatin therapy significantly reduced the length of stay for acute cardiac disease hospitalisations and revascularisation procedures.[72] Cost savings from reduction in healthcare use offset therapy cost by 88% with the effective cost of simvastatin estimated to be $US528 per patient or $US0.28 per day.

It should be pointed out that the 4S study population was at extremely high risk for CHD and atypical of the US heart disease at-risk population. The 4S study excluded patients with LDL cholesterol levels below 3.9 mmol/L (150 mg/dl) and had an average patient LDL cholesterol level of 4.9 mmol/L (188 mg/dl). Only 8% of the adult US population falling within the NCEP heart disease at-risk guidelines for cholesterol lowering are at high enough risk to meet the 4S study entry criteria. Moreover, the levels of use for CHD risk reduction interventions, such as revascularisation procedures, aspirin, β-blockers and ACE inhibitors, were substantially lower in the 4S study than has been observed in other statin clinical trials for secondary disease prevention.

Ashraf et al.[64] evaluated the cost effectiveness of pravastatin in secondary prevention of CHD. The analysis used actual clinical outcome data from 2 placebo-controlled pravastatin atherosclerotic plaque regression studies (PLAC studies) of patients with pre-existing heart disease and moderately elevated cholesterol levels [LDL threshold level of 3.4 mmol/L (130 mg/dl), average LDL level of 4.1 mmol/L (160 mg/dl)]. These regression trials found a 60% reduction in rates of MI over an average of 2.3 years of follow-up in 445 male patients. The analytical perspective was societal, but indirect costs (e.g. employer productivity losses) were not included. The analysis assumed a therapy initiation and monitoring cost of roughly $US1 per day, used FHS data to project the risk of mortality for the 10 years subsequent to MI and an expert panel of cardiologists to augment the literature-based medical care model.

For the base case, where patients were assumed to maintain pravastatin treatment only during the 3 years of study follow-up, Ashraf et al.[64] found costs per YLS of $US12 665, $US9368 and $US7124, respectively, for patients with 1, 2 and 3 additional CHD risk factors. In a sensitivity analysis, projecting the benefits of pravastatin to 10 years of treatment, the cost per YLS ranged from $US5500 to $US9600. The analysis concluded that pravastatin treatment was highly cost effective in secondary prevention of CHD.

A cost-effectiveness study using the 4S study projected to the US medical care system reported that the cost per YLS for simvastatin was $US13 967 for men and $US26 015 for women.[70] This is approximately double the baseline cost per YLS estimated by Ashraf et al.[64] for pravastatin in secondary disease. This is somewhat surprising since the baseline LDL cholesterol level in the pravastatin PLAC study population [4.1 mmol/L (160 mg/dl)] was lower than the baseline level in the simvastatin 4S study [4.9 mmol/L (188 mg/dl)]. Moreover, in addition to statin therapy, patients in the PLAC study received more aggressive surgical and medical treatment than the 4S patients.

Table IV. Five-year cardiovascular disease costs avoided per 1000 patients treated with pravastatin (results[25] and economic analysis[64] of the LIPID study)

Event	Events avoided per 1000 patients[25]	Average medical cost per event[64] ($US)	Acute medical savings ($US) [1998 values]
Death	32.34	16 376	529 583
MI	29.31	24 176	708 579
CABG	27.19	55 544	1 510 126
PTCA	12.69	18 868	239 391
Unstable angina pectoris	39.00	27 520	1 073 280
Stroke/TIA	8.62	20 945	180 510
Total	**149.14**		**4 241 469**

CABG = coronary artery bypass graft; **MI** = myocardial infarction; **PTCA** = percutaneaous transluminal angioplasty; **TIA** = transient ischaemic attack.

The cost-effectiveness ratio of simvastatin in the Swedish health system has also been reported based on 4S data, with a cost-effectiveness ratio of $US7500/YLS (1995 values).[73] This more favourable result derives primarily from the use of lower medication prices than those prevailing in the US.

The CARE and LIPID data permit reliable evaluation of the cost effectiveness of pravastatin for the vast majority of CHD patients, including those with pretreatment LDL cholesterol levels as low as 3.0 mmol/L (115 mg/dl) [table I]. Preliminary results of the cost-effectiveness analysis of the CARE and LIPID study data were not available at the time of writing. However, a highly favourable cost-effectiveness ratio is evident since significant reductions (24 to 30%) in the recurrent CHD rate and coronary revascularisation rate were observed in the CARE and LIPID studies, and a 23% reduction in mortality was observed in the larger LIPID study.

Daily net costs of $US0.13 for pravastatin (based on the US average wholesale price of 40mg pravastatin minus 15% price discount and average CHD medical care costs avoided in the study) and pravastatin cost-effectiveness estimates of less than $US5000 per YLS can be extrapolated; calculations are based on the secondary cost of CHD care (table IV) and the risk reduction in the CARE trial.[24] Notably, because of the low lipid thresholds in the CARE study, these favourable costs and cost-effectiveness ratios would apply to essentially the entire US population at risk for CHD because of pre-existing disease. This encompasses more than 6 million Americans.

Recent preliminary data released from the LIPID trial on pravastatin for an even broader segment of secondary prevention patients imply even more favourable economic results.[25] Extrapolating this preliminary clinical data using previously published US cardiovascular treatment cost estimates,[64] the average 5-year medical care savings from avoided CHD events using pravastatin for secondary disease prevention are estimated to be $US4.2 million per 1000 patients over 5 years or $US2.32 per patient per day. Since the US price of pravastatin (40mg) as discounted to many government and managed-care payers is at or below this cost level, many health plans will actually save net treatment costs (in addition to saving lives) by putting patients with pre-existing heart disease on pravastatin.

Despite the limited number of secondary prevention studies published so far, aggressive secondary prevention programmes using those HMG-CoA reductase inhibitors that have proven outcome benefits within specific populations such as pravastatin or simvastatin appear to be both clinically and economically justified. Since the cost effectiveness of these agents vary for patients of differing ages, pretreatment cholesterol levels, durations of treatment and CHD risks, future analyses should consider these factors simultaneously in order to fully define optimum individual treatment.

Indirect economic benefits, such as gain in productivity due to averted coronary events, as well as costs of treating drug-related adverse effects, should be taken into account in future analyses. Since agents within the same class differ in potency, cost, adverse effect and drug interaction profiles, clinical efficacy such as reduction in incidence in CHD and progression of atherosclerosis and possibly in their mechanisms of action, cost-effectiveness data for each agent is unlikely to be applicable to another lipid-lowering agent within the same class.[58,74-77]

4. Cost Effectiveness of Dietary Intervention

High fat/high caloric fat diet is the likely primary cause of hyperlipidaemia in the general population. Modification of plasma lipids can alter the progression of CHD.[15,78,79] Cholesterol lowering through dietary means has been widely adopted by clinicians as the initial mode of intervention in individuals with elevated serum cholesterol levels. Currently, dietary therapy such as a step I or step II diet is recommended by the NCEP[27] for individuals who have elevated cholesterol levels but are otherwise at low risk for CHD, such as young adults or premenopausal women. Step II diets are also recommended for secondary prevention in individuals with LDL cholesterol levels >2.6 mmol/L (>100 mg/dl), while drug therapy is reserved for those who have failed an adequate trial of dietary therapy.[27]

While it seems reasonable to assume that dietary therapy is effective over the longer term, data on the clinical feasibility, efficacy and cost effectiveness of step I and II diets are lacking. To date, no studies have proven the benefits of dietary monotherapy in terms of survival improvement. Few prospective studies have evaluated the effects of dietary intervention on cholesterol level and CHD event reduction.

The Leiden trial[78] and the Lifestyle Heart Trial[79] demonstrated favourable changes in serum lipids and coronary angiographies; however, the study diets were restrictive and of limited practicality. The St. Thomas' Atherosclerosis Regression Study (STARS)[15] evaluated the effect of a more practical lipid-lowering diet on lipids and coronary events. With frequent dietary counselling and encouragement, significant reduction in LDL cholesterol levels (16.2%), cardiac events and coronary atherosclerosis were observed in the 3-year follow-up period. Significant reduction in CHD mortality was not observed in the study.

The Cholesterol-Lowering Intervention Program (CLIP)[80] evaluated the clinical feasibility and efficacy of a step I diet in patients who were not taking lipid-lowering medications. Of three models studied, the greatest reduction in serum cholesterol level (8%) occurred in the nutritional centre model. Cholesterol level response was positively related to the length of follow-up. Approximately 42% of the patients who were referred to the nutritional centre model refused to participate. These results suggested that dietary therapy is inferior to drug therapy in CHD risk reduction and considerable patient variability exists in the efficacy of dietary intervention.

Cholesterol level reduction achieved by diet ranges from 5 to 15% and factors such as compliance and motivation of the patient, length of follow-up and amount of contact time between patient and nutritional counsellor are major determinants of success. Although one might assume that dietary therapy is more cost effective than drug therapy, this may not be true when one considers the additional personnel costs and office visit costs and more importantly, additional medical costs involved secondary to the suboptimal response achieved by dietary therapy. Impairment in quality of life associated with strict dietary regimens will also reduce the cost effectiveness of dietary therapy. Despite the current recommendations by the NCEP, evidence from recent statin clinical outcome studies underscore the need for early and aggressive initiation of drug therapy in individuals who have elevated cholesterol levels or in individuals who have CHD with LDL cholesterol levels >2.6 mmol/L (>100 mg/dl) since the response to step I and step II diets are often inadequate in achieving the desired LDL goal, and the CHD event risk reduction with dietary therapy is modest in any case.

5. Differences in Cost Effectiveness between Primary and Secondary Prevention Programmes

In contrast to other diseases such as infections or malignant disorders, lipid-lowering programmes for secondary prevention are generally more cost effective than for primary prevention when the same strategies are being applied to a population with similar CHD risk factors. In a study conducted by Goldman et al.[42] (discussed in sections 2 and 3), the cost-effectiveness ratio of primary prevention with lovastatin in high risk men ranged from $US41 580 to $US56 980/YLS, but was <$US29 400/YLS when the drug was used for secondary prevention.

Treatment for secondary prevention is more cost effective than for primary prevention because individuals with established CHD in general are at higher risk for recurrent coronary events and, therefore, more cost savings can be accrued from the cardiac disease avoided at similar costs of treatment.[8]

For example, using US cardiovascular treatment costs, primary prevention with pravastatin in the WOSCOPS study would have avoided $US1.04 in cardiovascular treatment costs per patient per day;[46] secondary prevention in the LIPID study would have avoided $US2.32 per patient per day (see table IV and section 3). Given the current US price of pravastatin as discounted to government and managed-care payers, secondary prevention with pravastatin results in medical care savings. Primary prevention with pravastatin increases direct medical treatment costs approximately $US1 per day per patient at the mean WOSCOPS CHD risk level.

However, the level of CHD risk among individuals receiving primary prevention may overlap with that among those receiving secondary prevention. Diabetics have as great a risk for CHD as patients who have already experienced symptomatic CHD.[81] In statin clinical trials, patients appear to benefit by similar relative amounts (20 to 40% event risk reduction) regardless of underlying absolute CHD risk levels (due to differences in age, gender, smoking, diabetes, hypertension, obesity, etc.). Particularly in light of the results of the WOSCOPS, CARE and LIPID pravastatin study results, the concept of who needs risk reduction through statin therapy should be reconsidered. The focus should be moved towards reducing the risk

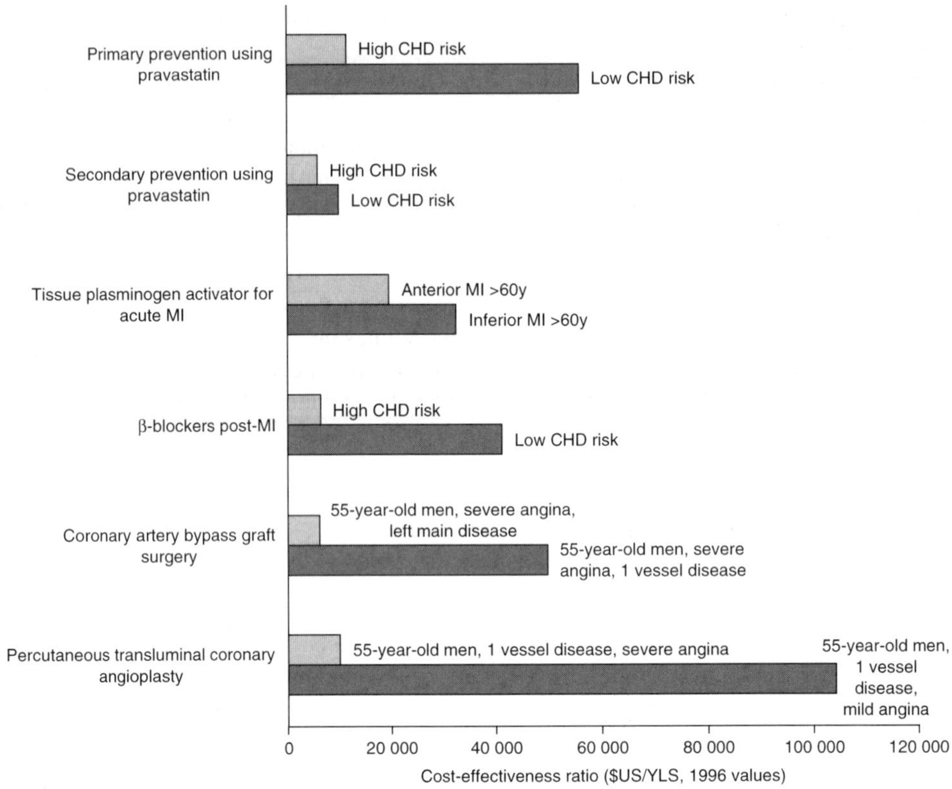

Fig. 1. Comparative cost effectiveness of different medical strategies for the management of coronary heart disease (CHD). Cost-effectiveness ratios adapted from references.[48,51,64,83-85]
MI = myocardial infarction; **YLS** = year of life saved.

of cardiovascular events in patients at highest risk (regardless of whether cholesterol is the most important risk factor for any given patient) and towards consideration of which therapy can accomplish the risk reduction goal in a cost-effective manner.

6. Comparative Cost Effectiveness of Primary and Secondary Prevention of CHD with Other Well-Accepted Medical Strategies

Lipid medications are perceived by many healthcare administrators to be unnecessarily expensive frills.[82] Fully-compliant use of these medications occurs in less than 10% of US patients for whom they are indicated. The two main arguments against the use of statins in the past were that they had not demonstrated outcome results and that they were too expensive. Recent clinical trials show that primary and secondary prevention of CHD in all high risk and many moderate risk patients using HMG-CoA reductase inhibitors, particularly pravastatin, compare favourably with other well-accepted medical interventions for cardiovascular disease such as coronary bypass graft surgery or percutaneous transluminal coronary angioplasty (fig. 1).[50,83-86] While differences in methodology and data reliability make comparisons across studies difficult, the cost effectiveness of cholesterol lowering for primary and secondary prevention of

CHD is also comparable to other commonly used noncardiovascular strategies such as haemodialysis or breast cancer screening.[51,87,88]

7. Limitations and Uncertainties of Current Pharmacoeconomic Studies

Although numerous pharmacoeconomic analyses have been performed to assess the economic benefits of lipid-lowering therapy, cost-effectiveness information is still limited in certain subgroups of patients such as female patients, especially those who are receiving hormonal replacement therapy, elderly patients aged >75 years, adults aged <35 years or those with concomitant hypertriglyceridemia or low HDL cholesterol levels.

Most available clinical studies either completely exclude or include very small numbers of these types of patients, preventing subgroup analysis. However, the CARE, LIPID, 4S and AFCAPS/ TexCAPS studies did show significant therapeutic efficacy6 in women, the elderly and other subgroups of patients that was at least as good as that in the overall study populations. At this point, there is no reason to assume that the clinical trial benefits that have been demonstrated for a given therapy are not generalisable to other population subgroups, at least for that therapy.

As mentioned earlier, pharmacoeconomic studies that have analysed the cost effectiveness of lipid-lowering agents in the context of one country's healthcare system may not be applicable to another system. International extrapolation of these study results is difficult since health resource costs and healthcare use rates vary between countries and, therefore, the cost effectiveness of these agents in different countries can vary significantly. This is not as much of a problem with primary prevention studies as with secondary prevention studies, since health system variation is likely to have a much more pronounced impact on the course of CHD after it becomes a recognised disease than before.

Comparison of the published cost-effectiveness studies is also confounded by evaluation of populations with different characteristics, different CHD risk levels, from different perspectives and at various lengths of treatment duration. Moreover, definitions of net costs in these studies also differ significantly: some studies did not consider indirect costs while others included the non-CHD medical costs. Adverse event treatment costs for statins have consistently been shown in clinical trials thus far to be negligible. However, since statins differ in their susceptibility for interactions with other medications due to differences in their metabolic pathways, and since these interactions are more likely to be aggressively monitored and corrected in clinical trials than in actual practice, real-world differences in adverse events may differ from those reported in clinical trials.[76,89-92] Future analyses comparing different classes of lipid medications should also consistently consider compliance and adverse effect treatment costs and indirect savings associated with labour and productivity gain secondary to disease avoided.

Incorporation of QOL analysis in the estimate would also be beneficial since some forms of lipid therapy may adversely affect the quality of life of asymptomatic patients but at the same time improve the quality of life of symptomatic patients by delaying CHD morbidity. Development of reliable tools to measure health-related quality of life will facilitate research in this area.

Finally, inclusion of non-CHD medical costs in the cost-effectiveness estimate is not warranted except where the analysis is done from a medical care payer perspective.

8. Conclusion

Pharmacoeconomic studies affect real world medical choices. Head-to-head clinical comparison of survival outcomes with all, or even several, of the lipid-lowering agents for all population subgroups is not financially realistic. Healthcare decision-makers will have to make policy choices about the appropriate use of lipid therapy in patient subgroups for whom only incomplete data are available.

At this point in our clinical and economic understanding of lipid therapy, the main point that should be stressed is that statins – particularly pravastatin for primary and secondary prevention, simvastatin for secondary prevention and lovastatin for primary prevention – have been shown to reduce CHD in a cost-effective fashion. The LIPID study showed that for most patients at risk for secondary disease, pravastatin will actually save direct medical treatment costs when US prices and medical interventions are used in the analysis.

The other key conclusion is that the notion of a 'class effect' for lipid medications (and dietary interventions) has not been proven. Some data suggest that the CHD risk reduction produced by pravastatin is greater than that predicted by estimates based on lipid-lowering and epidemiological data (section 2.4.2). Better outcomes data are required to determine whether the same is true of other statins and lipid treatments. The only clinical trial of niacin demonstrating outcome benefits found a substantially weaker reduction in CHD events than the statin results after 6 years of follow-up, even though niacin is more potent at lowering LDL and raising HDL cholesterol levels than typical statin dosages.[10] There is recent clinical speculation that niacin's negative impact on homocysteine levels may offset some of its lipid benefits in preventing CHD.

Particularly in the cardiology field, there have been numerous examples of medications, many still in use, that were included in standard medical practice because of short-term clinical data on intermediate clinical measures (such as blood tests, blood pressure readings, ECGs, lipid values, etc.) but later, common uses of these medications were found to be inappropriate, risky, harmful or sometimes fatal. These medications include fenfluramine-phentermine, non-potassium-sparing diuretics, short-acting calcium channel blockers, prophylactic lidocaine and type Ic anti-arrhythmics.[93-100]

Net clinical benefit of lipid lowering has been demonstrated for several agents, including colestyramine, niacin, gemfibrozil, pravastatin, lovastatin and simvastatin. Of these, colestyramine and niacin have substantial tolerance and compliance concerns,[10,13,14] while gemfibrozil may have safety concerns at high therapeutic doses.[18] The safety and tolerability evidence on statin therapy is overwhelmingly favourable.

The evidence that has accumulated thus far suggests not all lipid therapy is the same and that not all of the statins are identical in their effectiveness on clinical outcomes (as opposed to their lipid effects). For example, because of its large scope, there was a sizable number of CARE patients who would have met the study entry criteria for the 4S study. In that subset of CARE patients, the reduction in coronary events was 43%, which compares favourably to the overall 4S event reduction of 37%. This is notable since the upper study entry LDL cholesterol level cutoff criterion for the CARE study was 4.5 mmol/L (175 mg/dl) while the average LDL cholesterol level for 4S patients was 4.8 mmol/L (188 mg/dl). The use of additional CHD risk reduction medication was equivalent or higher in the CARE trial than in the 4S study (use of aspirin: 83 *vs* 37%, β-blockers: 40 *vs* 57%, nitrates: 33 *vs* 33%, calcium channel blockers: 39

vs 31%, ACE inhibitors: 15% *vs* not reported), and the rate of revascularisation procedures was also substantially higher in the CARE trial than in the 4S. All of these factors would bias in favour of a greater risk reduction for simvastatin in 4S than for pravastatin in the CARE subgroup meeting the 4S study entry criteria, but the event risk reduction point estimate was higher in the CARE study than in the 4S study. Moreover, since the 4S study achieved a 35% reduction in LDL cholesterol levels and an 8% increase in HDL cholesterol levels while the LDL effect of pravastatin in CARE was a reduction of 28% and the HDL effect was an increase of 5%, differential lipid changes between the 2 statin drugs did not seem to reflect the entire difference in clinical effectiveness.

It is also noteworthy that while atherosclerotic plaque regression studies have been conducted and reported for all of the statins except cerivastatin and atorvastatin, and while more than 1000 patient years of follow-up exist for each of these other statins, only pravastatin has shown significant reductions in coronary events in the context of such relatively small sample/short term follow-up clinical trials of quantitative disease regression. Given this evidence, it is important to ask not only how are some statins able to achieve significant clinical event reductions, but also why have other statins failed to demonstrate these benefits in similar studies.

Measuring the cost and the effectiveness of these agents simultaneously in head-to-head pharmacoeconomic outcomes studies (using only active comparators for those patients where proven therapy indications are available) would dramatically enhance therapeutic decision-making. It is time to rethink the research designs for undertaking randomised trials so as to rigorously assess the relative cost effectiveness of alternative lipid therapies. Ideally, one would like to see clinical outcomes, pharmacoeconomic and survival comparisons for all of the statins, niacin, resins, fibrates and combination therapies in a randomised trial. The cost of such a study would be in the hundreds of millions of dollars. No pharmaceutical company, health plan or single government agency could be expected to cover the enormous costs of such a study by themselves. However, such a study would be easily justified to society.

For example, since pravastatin has been shown to reduce cardiovascular mortality by 24% and since more than 740 000 US patients die from heart disease each year, using pravastatin in all patients who are at high risk for CHD could potentially save over 170 000 lives in the US annually.[4,25] Even if each of these lives were worth only $US10 000, a billion dollar study that would convincingly prove which lipid treatment strategy should be implemented for all population subgroups would pay for itself in 1 year. If done in the US, such a study would have to involve the cooperation of several health plans and pharmaceutical companies. Much of the expensive laboratory testing and other clinical protocols including treatment blinding associated with typical clinical trials would not be acceptable for such a study, since these items would raise the study costs to prohibitive levels, and would make the study less accurate in reflecting real-world medical decision-making.

The cost effectiveness of primary and secondary prevention of CHD using the proven evidence for pravastatin, lovastatin and simvastatin also compares favourably with other medical strategies for cardiovascular disease. Primary prevention using pravastatin is cost effective in most high risk patients, with cost effectiveness improving in individuals as the risk for CHD increases. On the other hand, pravastatin therapy for secondary prevention is highly cost effective in all patients with pre-existing disease and may be cost saving in many patients (e.g.

patients meeting the LIPID study entry criteria), with savings due to avoided disease offsetting medication cost by over 100%.

Pravastatin is the only lipid medication that has proven survival benefits for both primary and secondary disease prevention. Other statins and lipid-lowering agents may enhance survival in all patients at risk for CHD, but this remains to be rigorously demonstrated. Policy-makers today must weigh the evidence of proven survival benefits with pravastatin against price or lipid modification potency considerations for other lipid agents. Is a 20% drug price differential worth switching to a drug with unproven clinical outcomes? How does one compare a drug that has greater ability to lower LDL cholesterol levels with no evidence of disease reduction against a less potent drug that has proven its ability to reduce cardiovascular disease and mortality?

In order to maximise the therapeutic outcomes while minimising the financial burden of CHD, revision of the current NCEP treatment guidelines based on the new clinical and pharmacoeconomic evidence is necessary. A cost-effective cholesterol intervention programme should use HMG-CoA reductase inhibitors such as pravastatin as preferred agents for primary and secondary prevention of CHD in patients with elevated cholesterol and normal triglycerides levels, or other substantial risks for CHD.

Moreover, more aggressive statin treatment should also be implemented in patients with evident CHD. Furthermore, population-wide cholesterol lowering by dietary therapy may also be a cost-effective strategy to lower the national CHD mortality rate and should be encouraged through public health and public information policies.[101] A gradual and slow downward shift in the average population LDL cholesterol levels brought about through low-cost mass media and public education campaigns, particularly when effectively targeted at children and others whose dietary behaviour is relatively susceptible to modification, may achieve large long term societal payoffs in reducing coronary disease.[102] However, targeted cholesterol lowering by diet monotherapy alone is no longer optimal for many patients with identified CHD or high levels of CHD risk. Early and aggressive initiation of statin therapy is clinically necessary in most individuals with known CHD risk.

Such interventions can now be concluded to be cost effective as well. Based on US medical price levels and the available clinical trial data on statins, it will be cost effective (e.g. cost less than $US50 000/YLS) to intervene on any patient with annual CHD risk exceeding 1%. This includes all patients with pre-existing CHD and many more primary prevention patients than are currently contemplated by the NCEP treatment guidelines. Achieving such a goal will require enormous changes in patient education, clinical perspective, healthcare practice and healthcare finances. But any proven opportunity for saving the lives of 25% of those dying from cardiovascular disease each year deserves to be considered with the utmost seriousness and urgency.

References

1. Gillium RF. Trends in acute myocardial infarction and coronary heart disease death in the United States. J Am Coll Cardiol 1993; 23: 1273-7
2. Goldman L, Cook F. The decline in ischemic heart disease mortality rates: an analysis of the comparative effects of medical interventions and changes in lifestyle. Ann Intern Med 1984; 101: 825-36
3. Sytokwski PA, Kannel WB, Agostino RB. Changes in risk factor and the decline in mortality from cardiovascular disease: The Framingham Heart Study. N Engl J Med 1990; 322: 1635-41
4. American Heart Association. 1998 Heart and stroke statistical update. Dallas (TX): American Heart Association, 1988
5. Wittels EH, Hay JW, Gotto AM. Medical costs of coronary artery disease. Am J Cardiol 1990; 65: 432-40

6. Castelli WP, Anderson KM, Wilson PW, et al. Lipids and risk of coronary heart disease: The Framingham Study. Ann Epidemiol 1992; 2: 23-8
7. Levy D, Wilson WF, Anderson KM, et al. Stratifying the patient at risk from coronary disease: new insights from the Framingham heart study. Am Heart J 1990; 119: 712-7
8. Wong ND, Wilson PW, Kannel WB. Serum cholesterol as a prognostic factor after myocardial infarction: The Framingham Study. Ann Intern Med 1991; 115: 687-93
9. Stamler J, Wentworth D, Neaton JD. Is the relationship between serum cholesterol and risk of premature death from coronary heart disease continuous and graded? JAMA 1986; 256: 2823-8
10. Canner PL, Berge KG, Wenger NK, et al. Fifteen year mortality in Coronary Drug Project Research Group: long-term benefit with niacin. J Am Coll Cardiol 1986; 8: 1245-55
11. Blankenhorn DW, Nessim SA, Johnson RL, et al. Beneficial effects of combined colestipol-niacin therapy on coronary atherosclerosis and coronary venous bypass grafts. JAMA 1987; 257: 3233-40
12. Multiple Risk Factor Intervention Trial Research Group. Relationship between baseline risk factors and coronary heart disease and total mortality in the multiple risk factor intervention trial. Prev Med 1986; 15: 254-73
13. Lipid Research Clinics Program. The Lipid Research Clinics Coronary Primary Prevention Trials Results. I: reduction in incidence of coronary heart disease. JAMA 1984; 251: 351-64
14. Lipid Research Clinics Program. The Lipid Research Clinical Coronary Primary Prevention Trials Results. II: the relationship of reduction in incidence of coronary heart disease to cholesterol-lowering. JAMA 1984; 251: 365-74
15. Watts GF, Lewis B, Brunt JN, et al. Effects on coronary artery disease of lipid-lowering diet, or diet plus cholestyramine, in the St. Thomas' Atherosclerosis Regression Study (STARS). Lancet 1992; 339: 563-9
16. Brown G, Albers JJ, Fisher LD, et al. Regression of coronary artery disease as a result of intensive lipid lowering therapy in men with high levels of apolipoprotein B. N Engl J Med 1990; 323: 1289-98
17. Buchwald H, Varco RL, Matts JP, et al. Effect of partial ileal bypass surgery on mortality and morbidity from coronary heart disease in patients with hypercholesterolemia. N Engl J Med 1990; 323: 946-66
18. Frick MH, Elo O, Haapa K, et al. Helsinki Heart Study: primary prevention trial with gemfibrozil in middle-aged men with dyslipidemia. Safety of treatment, changes in risk factors and incidence of coronary heart disease. N Engl J Med 1987; 317: 1237-45
19. Shepherd J, Cobbe SM, Ford I, et al. Prevention of coronary heart disease with pravastatin in men with hypercholesterolemia. N Engl J Med 1995; 333: 1301-7
20. Downs JR, Clearfield M, Weiss S, AFCAPS/TexCAPS Research Group, et al. Primary prevention of acute coronary events with lovastatin in men and women with average cholesterol levels: results of AFCAPS/TexCAPS. JAMA 1998; 279 (20): 1615-22
21. Scandinavian Simvastatin Survival Study Group. Randomized trial of cholesterol lowering in 4444 patients with coronary heart disease: the Scandinavian Simvastatin Survival Study. Lancet 1994; 344: 1383-9
22. Pitt B, Mancini J, Ellis SG, et al. Pravastatin limitation of atherosclerosis in the coronary arteries (PLAC-I): reduction in atherosclerosis progression and clinical events. J Am Coll Cardiol 1995; 26: 1133-9
23. Crouse JB, Byington RP, Bond MG, et al. Pravastatin, lipids, and atherosclerosis in the carotid arteries (PLAC-II). Am J Cardiol 1995; 75: 455-9
24. Sacks FM, Pfeffer MA, Moye LA, et al. The effect of pravastatin on coronary events after myocardial infarction in patients with average cholesterol levels. N Engl J Med 1996; 335: 1001-9
25. The Long-Term Intervention with Pravastatin in Ischaemic Disease (LIPID) Study Group. Prevention of cardiovascular events and death with pravastatin in patients with coronary heart disease and a broad range of initial cholesterol levels. N Engl J Med 1998; 339: 1349-57
26. Byington RP, Jukema JW, Salonen JT, et al. Reduction in cardiovascular events during pravastatin therapy: pooled analysis of clinical events of the pravastatin atherosclerosis intervention program. Circulation 1995; 92: 2419-25
27. Expert Panel on Detection, Evaluation and Treatment of High Blood Cholesterol in Adults. Summary of the second report of the National Cholesterol Education Program (NCEP) Expert Panel on Detection, Evaluation and Treatment of High Blood Cholesterol in Adults. JAMA 1993; 269 (23): 3015-23
28. Freund D, Dittus R. Principles of pharmacoeconomic evaluation of drug therapy. Pharmacoeconomics 1992; 1 (1): 20-32
29. Weinstein M, Stason W. Foundations of cost effectiveness analysis for health and medical practices. N Engl J Med 1977; 296 (13): 716-21
30. O'Brien B, Rushby J. Outcome assessment in cardiovascular cost-benefit studies. Am Heart J 1990; 119: 740-8
31. Kupersmith J, Helmes-Rovner M, Hogan A, et al. Cost-effectiveness analysis in heart disease. Pt I: general principles. Prog Cardiovasc Dis 1994; 37 (3): 161-84
32. Hay J. Reporting pharmacoeconomic model results. Value Health 1998; 1 (3): 187-93
33. Hay JW, Wittels EH, Gotto AM. An economic evaluation of lovastatin for cholesterol lowering and coronary artery disease reduction. Am J Cardiol 1991; 67: 789-96
34. Sempos CT, Cleeman JI, Carroll MD, et al. Prevalence of high blood cholesterol among U.S. adults: an update based on guidelines from the second report of the national cholesterol education program adult treatment panel. JAMA 1993; 269: 3009-14
35. Kinosian BP, Eisenberg JM. Cutting into cholesterol: cost-effective alternatives for treating hypercholesterolemia. JAMA 1988; 259: 2249-54
36. Weinstein MC, Stason WB. Cost-effectiveness of interventions to prevent or treat coronary heart disease. Ann Rev Public Health 1985; 6: 41-63
37. Schulman KA, Kinosian B, Jacobson TA, et al. Reducing high blood cholesterol level with drugs: cost-effectiveness of pharmacologic management. JAMA 1990; 264: 3025-33

38. Oster G, Epstein AM. Cost-effectiveness of antihyperlipidemic therapy in the prevention of coronary heart disease: the case of cholestyramine. JAMA 1987; 258: 2381-7
39. Martens LL, Rutten FF, Erkelens W, et al. Clinical benefits and cost-effectiveness of lowering serum cholesterol levels: the case of simvastatin and cholestyramine in the Netherlands. Am J Cardiol 1990; 65: 27F-32F
40. Martens LL, Rutten FF. Cost effectiveness of cholesterol-lowering therapy in the Netherlands. Am J Med 1989; 87 Suppl. 4A: 54S-8S
41. Kelley MD. Hypercholesterolemia: the cost of treatment in perspective. South Med J 1990; 83 (12): 1421-5
42. Goldman P, Lee TH, Weinstein MC, Goldman PA, et al. Cost-effectiveness of HMG-CoA reductase inhibition for primary and secondary prevention of coronary heart disease. JAMA 1991; 265: 1145-51
43. Hamilton VH, Racicot FE, Zowall H, et al. The cost-effectiveness of HMG-CoA reductase inhibitors to prevent coronary heart disease. JAMA 1995; 273: 1032-8
44. Martens LL, Guibert R. Cost-effectiveness analysis of lipid modifying therapy in Canada: comparison of HMG-CoA reductase inhibitors in the primary prevention of coronary heart disease. Clin Ther 1994; 16 (6): 1052-62
45. WOSCOPS Economic Analysis Group. The West of Scotland Coronary Prevention Study: weighing the cost and benefits of primary prevention with pravastatin. BMJ 1997; 315: 1577-82
46. Hay J, Lapuerta P, Yuan Y, et al. Pravastatin cost-effectiveness for primary prevention of cardiovascular disease in the United States [abstract]. American Heart Association 70th Scientific Session; 1997 Nov; Orlando
47. Johannesson M, Borgquist L, Jonsson B, et al. The cost effectiveness of lipid lowering in Swedish primary health care. J Intern Med 1996; 240: 23-9
48. Drummond MF, O'Brien B, Stoddart GL, et al. Methods for economic evaluation of health care programmes. 2nd ed. London: Oxford University Press, 1997
49. Laupacis A, Feeny D, Detsky AS, et al. How attractive does a new technology have to be to warrant adoption and utilization? Tentative guidelines for using clinical and economic evaluations. Can Med Assoc J 1992; 146 (4): 473-81
50. Mark DB, Hlatky MA, Califf RM, et al. Cost effectiveness of thrombolytic therapy with tissue plasminogen activator as compared with streptokinase for acute myocardial infarction. N Engl J Med 1995; 332: 1418-24
51. Tengs TO, Adams ME, Pliskin JS, et al. Five hundred life-saving interventions and their cost-effectiveness. Risk Anal 1995; 15 (3): 369-90
52. Dorr AE, Gundersen K, Schneider JC, et al. Colestipol hydrochloride in hypercholesterolemic patients: effect on serum cholesterol and mortality. J Chronic Dis 1978; 31: 5-14
53. Kirby RW, Anderson JW, Sieling B. Oat bran intake selectively lowers serum low-density lipoprotein cholesterol concentrations. Am J Clin Nutr 1981; 34: 824-9
54. Syam S, Fifer SK. Gemfibrozil cost-benefit study: targeting subgroups for effective hyperlipidemia drug therapy. Drugs 1990; 40 Suppl. 1: 42-52
55. Perrealt S, Hamilton VH, Lavoie F, et al. A head-to-head comparison of the cost effectiveness of HMG-CoA reductase inhibitors and fibrates in different types of primary hyperlipidemia. Cardiovasc Drugs Ther 1996; 10: 787-94
56. Bakker-Arkema RG, Davidson MH, Goldstein RJ, et al. Efficacy and safety of a new HMG-CoA reductase inhibitor, atorvastatin, in patients with hypertriglyceridemia. JAMA 1996; 275: 128-33
57. Bischoff H, Angerbauer R, Bender J, et al. Cerivastatin: pharmacology of a novel synthetic and highly active HMG-CoA reductase inhibitor. Atherosclerosis 1997; 135 (1): 119-30
58. Rosenson RS, Tangney CC. Antiatherothrombotic properties of statins: implications for cardiovascular event reduction. JAMA 1998; 279: 1643-50
59. Pilote L, Granger C, Armstrong PW, et al. Differences in the treatment of myocardial infarction between the United States and Canada. Med Care 1995; 33 (6): 598-610
60. Blum CB. Comparison of properties of four inhibitors of 3-hydroxy-3-methylglutaryl-conenzyme A reductase. Am J Cardiol 1994; 73: 3D-11D
61. Conti CR. Economics of lipid lowering with HMG-CoA reductase inhibitors [letter]. Clin Cardiol 1995; 18: 60
62. Roberts WC. Retail costs of the statin lipid-lowering drugs [editorial]. Am J Cardiol 1994; 74: 1181
63. Gotto AM, Hay JW. Cost of lipid-lowering statin drugs [letter]. Am J Cardiol 1996; 77: 226
64. Ashraf T, Hay JW, Pitt B, et al. Cost-effectiveness of pravastatin in secondary prevention of coronary artery disease. Am J Cardiol 1996; 78: 409-14
65. Spearman ME, Summers K, Moore V, et al. Cost-effectiveness of initial therapy with 3-hydroxy-3-methylglutaryl coenzyme A reductase inhibitors to treat hypercholesterolemia in a primary care setting of a managed-care organization. Clin Ther 1997; 19: 582-602
66. Koren MJ, Smith DG, Hunninghake DB, et al. The cost of reaching National Cholesterol Education Program (NCEP) Goals in hypercholesterolaemic patients: a comparison of atorvastatin, simvastatin, lovastatin and fluvastatin. Pharmacoeconomics 1998; 14 (1): 59-70
67. American Heart Association Annual Meeting. Abstract; 1998 Nov; Dallas (TX)
68. Tyroler HA. Review of lipid-lowering clinical trials in relation to observational epidemiologic studies. Circulation 1987; 76: 515-22
69. Leaverton PE, Sorlie PD, Kleinman JC, et al. Representativeness of the Framingham risk model for coronary heart disease mortality: a comparison with a national cohort study. J Chronic Dis 1987; 40: 775-84
70. Johannesson M, Jonsson B, Kjeksjus J, et al. Cost effectiveness of simvastatin treatment to lower cholesterol levels in patients with coronary heart disease. N Engl J Med 1997; 336: 332-6
71. Reckless JP. The 4S study and its pharmacoeconomic implications. Pharmacoeconomics 1996; 9 (2): 101-5
72. Pedersen TR, Kjekshus J, Berg K, et al. Cholesterol lowering and the use of health care resources: results of the Scandinavian Simvastatin Survival Study. Circulation 1996; 93: 1796-802

73. Jonsson B, Johannesson M, Kjekshus J, et al. Cost-effectiveness of cholesterol lowering: results from the Scandinavian Simvastatin Survival Study (4S). Eur Heart J 1996; 17: 1001-7
74. West of Scotland Coronary Prevention Study Group. Influence of pravastatin and plasma lipids on clinical events in the West of Scotland Coronary Prevention Study. Circulation 1998; 97 (15): 1440-5
75. Pedersen TR, Olsson AG, Faergeman O, et al. Lipoprotein changes and reduction in the incidence of major coronary heart disease events in the Scandinavian Simvastatin Survival Study. Circulation 1998; 97 (15): 1453-60
76. Lennernas H, Fager G. Pharmacodynamics and pharmackinetics of the HMG-CoA reductase inhibitors: similarities and differences. Clin Pharmacokinet 1997; 32 (5): 403-25
77. Shepherd J, Park JS. Prevention of heart disease: is LDL reduction the outcome of choice? Value Health 1998; 1 (2): 120-4
78. Arntzenius AC, Kromhout D, Barth JD, et al. Diet, lipoproteins and the progression of coronary atherosclerosis. N Engl J Med 1985; 312: 805-11
79. Ornish D, Brown SE, Scherwitz LW, et al. Can lifestyle changes reverse coronary heart disease? Lancet 1990; 336: 129-33
80. Caggiula AW, Watson JE, Kuller LH, et al. Cholesterol-lowering intervention program: effect of the step I diet in community offices practices. Arch Intern Med 1996; 156: 1205-13
81. Haffner SM, Lehto S, Ronnemaa T, et al. Mortality from coronary heart disease in subjects with type 2 diabetes and in nondiabetic subjects with and without prior myocardial infarction. N Engl J Med 1998; 339 (4): 229-34
82. Bonnette J. Decision making in lipid therapy: a managed care perspective. Value Health. In press
83. Weinstein MC, Stason WB. Cost-effectiveness of coronary artery bypass surgery. Circulation 1982; 66 Suppl. III: 56-66
84. Wong JB, Sonnenberg FA, Salem DN, et al. Myocardial revascularization for chronic stable angina: analysis of the role of percutaneous transluminal coronary angioplasty based on data available in 1989. Ann Intern Med 1990; 113: 852-71
85. Goldman L, Sia SB, Cook EF, et al. Costs and effectiveness of routine therapy with long-term beta adrenergic antagonists after myocardial infarction. N Engl J Med 1988; 319: 152-7
86. Hlatky MA, Rogers WJ, Johnstone I, et al. Medical care costs and quality of life after randomization to coronary angioplasty or coronary bypass surgery. N Engl J Med 1997; 336: 92-9
87. Roberts SD, Maxwell DR, Gross TL. Cost-effective care of end-stage renal disease: a billion dollar question [editorial]. Ann Intern Med 1980; 92: 243
88. Garner TI, Dardis R. Cost-effectiveness analysis of end-stage renal disease treatments. Med Care 1987; 25: 25-34
89. White CM, Chow M. A review of HMG-CoA reductase inhibitors. Pharmacist 1998; 1: HS19-28
90. Boberg M, Angerbauer R, Fey P, et al. Metabolism of cerivastatin by human liver microsomes in vitro. Drug Metab Dispos 1997; 25 (3): 321-31
91. Neuvonen PJ, Kantola T, Kivisto K. Simvastatin but not pravastatin is very susceptible to interaction with the CYP3A4 inhibitor itraconazole. Clin Pharmacol Ther 1998; 63: 332-41
92. Kantola T, Kivisto K, Neuvonen P. Effect of itraconazole on pharmacokinetics of atorvastatin. Clin Pharmacol Ther 1998; 64: 58-65
93. Hoes AW, Grobbee DE, Lubsen J, et al. Diuretics, beta-blockers, and the risk for sudden cardiac death in hypertensive patients. Ann Intern Med 1995; 123: 481-7
94. Psaty BM, Heckbert SR, Koepsell TD, et al. The risk of myocardial infarction associated with antihypertensive drug therapies. JAMA 1996: 27; 620-5
95. Nattel S, Arenal A. Antiarrhythmic prophylaxis after acute myocardial infarction: is lidocaine still useful? Drugs 1993; 45 (1): 9-14
96. Hine LK, Laird N, Hewitt P, et al. Meta-analytic evidence against prophylactic use of lidocaine in acute myocardial infarction. Arch Intern Med 1989; 149: 2694-8
97. MacMahon S, Collins R, Peto R, et al. Effects of prophylactic lidocaine in suspected acute myocardial infarction: an overview of results from the randomized, controlled trials. JAMA 1988; 260: 1910-6
98. The Cardiac Arrhythmia Suppression Trial investigators. Preliminary report: effect of encainide and flecainide on mortality in a randomized trial of arrhythmia suppression after myocardial infarction. N Engl J Med 1989; 321 (6): 406-12
99. The Cardiac Arrhythmia Suppression Trial II investigators. Effect of the antiarrhythmic agent moricizine on survival after myocardial infarction. N Engl J Med 1992; 327 (4): 227-33
100. Connolly HM, Crary JL, Mcgoon MD, et al. Valvular heart disease associated with fenfluramine-phentermine. N Engl J Med 1997; 337 (9): 581-8
101. Goldman L, Weinstein MC, Williams LW. Relative impact of targeted versus population wide cholesterol interventions on the incidence of coronary artery disease: projections of the coronary heart disease policy model. Circulation 1989; 80: 254-60
102. Berwick DM, Cretin S, Keeler E. Cholesterol, children and heart disease: an analysis of alternatives. Pediatrics 1981; 68 (5): 721-30

Correspondence: Dr *Joel Hay*, Department of Pharmaceutical Economics and Policy, University of Southern California CHP 140, 1540 E. Alcazar St., Los Angeles CA 90033, USA.
E-mail: jhay@hsc.usc.edu

New Approaches to Coronary Heart Disease
Induction of Neovascularisation by Growth Factors

Thomas J. Stegmann

Department of Thoracic and Cardiovascular Surgery, Fulda Medical Center, Fulda, Germany

Coronary heart disease (CHD) is still one of the most common diseases in industrialised countries. 500 to 550 cases of myocardial infarction per 100 000 inhabitants occur from this disease every year in Europe; approximately 800 000 patients worldwide undergo bypass surgery each year and another 800 000 have the less invasive procedure balloon angioplasty (PTCA).[1] Additionally, about another 150 000 patients have CHD and are not candidates for either procedure because of a disadvantageous pattern of closure, or because of coronary arteries with diffuse atherosclerosis reaching out into the periphery.

Although the importance of new blood vessel formation and development – i.e. angiogenesis – in cancer has been well documented, the use of angiogenesis to restore blood flow to the ischaemic myocardium has so far received less attention. However, as shown by the extensive experimental research in this field and the recent attempts to treat human patients with peripheral or coronary atherosclerotic disease by induction of neo-angiogenesis, basic scientific as well as clinical research has now focused on this evolving new modality for treatment of cardiovascular disease.

1. Angiogenic Growth Factors

An entirely new therapeutic approach to atherosclerotic disease originated from the discovery of, and further research on, the so-called endothelial growth factors, especially those with angiogenic potency.[2-5] A number of naturally occurring growth factors can induce angiogenesis by stimulating endothelial cell growth, differentiation and migration. One of the polypeptides with endothelial mitogenic potency is vascular endothelial growth factor (VEGF), also known as vascular permeability factor.[6-8] Other widely studied growth factors include those in the fibroblast growth factor (FGF) family, especially FGF-1 (aFGF, acidic) and FGF-2 (bFGF, basic).[4,6] FGF, like VEGF, belongs to the group of heparin-binding growth factors (HBGF), and thus binds to heparin-like components of the extracellular matrix on the surface of endothelial and smooth muscle cells, thereby facilitating attachment of these growth factors to their high-affinity receptors.[7-9] Apart from their mitogenic stimulation of various types of cells, these factors are able to induce the differentiation of mesodermal tissue in the embryo, and to assist the differentiation and regeneration of neurones and the final stages of differentiation of skeletal muscle.[10] Other growth factors present in or near the vessel wall can also induce endothelial proliferation, such as transforming growth factor (TGF), hepatocyte growth factor and platelet-derived growth factor (PDGF).[11-13] The fundamental importance of the

Table I. General view of some well known heparin-binding growth factors with angiogenic efficacy

Growth factor	Endothelial cell receptor	Tissue distribution
FGF-1 (acidic)	FGFR-1, -2, -3, -4	Brain, heart, kidney, retina, etc.
FGF-2 (basic)	FGFR-1, -2	Brain, heart, kidney, retina, placenta, testes, etc.
FGF-4	FGFR-1, -2	Embryonic tissue
VEGF-A	VEGFR-1 (flt-1, fms) VEGFR-2 (kdr/flb-1)	Pituitary cells, monocytes, heart, lung, etc.
VEGF-B	Unknown	Heart, skeletal muscle, pancreas, etc.
VEGF-C	flt-4 (VEGFR-3/-2)	Heart, placenta, ovary, etc.

FGF = fibroblast growth factor; **FGFR** = FGF receptor; **VEGF** = vascular endothelial growth factor; **VEGFR** = VEGF receptor.

angiogenic growth factors is evident from the fact that the removal of, for example, the VEGF gene is lethal early in embryogenesis in animals (table I).[14]

Research in the field of angiogenesis started nearly 30 years ago, and was predominantly directed to the interaction of angiogenesis and tumour growth.[4,15] In 1971, Folkman published the hypothesis that tumours are angiogenesis-dependent.[15] In the 1970s it became possible to study regeneration and turnover rates of human endothelial cells in culture.[16] Subsequently, bioassays for angiogenesis were developed throughout that decade. In the 1980s, the isolation, characterisation and purification of the first growth factors with angiogenic potentiality were reported,[17-19] as was the discovery of inhibitors of angiogenesis.[20,21] The first translation of these laboratory findings to clinical application started in 1989 with the first treatment of haemangiomas in infants with interferon-α.[22] In the early 1990s came the discovery of a set of proteins – the so-called angiostatin and endostatin – so effective that they eradicated tumours in mice.[23]

Today, clinical applications of angiogenesis research are focused on three general topics: (i) antiangiogenic therapy (especially for tumours); (ii) prognostic markers in cancer patients; and (iii) angiogenic therapy (especially for ischaemic tissues). The first attempt at angiogenic therapy for human ischaemic peripheral vascular disease was the application of intra-arterial and intramuscular gene transfer of naked plasmid DNA encoding human VEGF in patients with severe vascular disease in the lower limbs.[24,25] The first report of angiogenic therapy of coronary heart disease in humans was published by our group in February 1998.[26]

2. Angiogenesis

In established blood vessels in mature organisms, the endothelial cells remain in a quiescent, nonproliferative state until stimulation of angiogenesis occurs by conditions such as wounding, inflammation, hypoxia or ischaemia. The formation of new vessels can be considered as the result of several processes: (i) dissolution of the matrix underlying the endothelial cell layer; (ii) migration, adhesion and proliferation of endothelial cells; (iii) formation of a new 3-dimensional tube, which then lengthens from its tip as circulation is re-established; and (iv) in larger vessels, vascular smooth muscle cells also migrate and adhere to the newly deposited matrix of the nascent vessel.[10] Angiogenic growth factors induce, promote or interfere with all these steps of angiogenesis.

In addition to their role in the initial development of the vascular system, angiogenic growth factors, like FGF and VEGF, and their receptors are expressed by endothelial cells in capillaries sprouting out from established vessels in response to pathological conditions. Expression of receptors for FGF and VEGF varies according to the vascular bed – with little or no expression in the normal myocardium – and can be altered by ischaemia.[12,13] Reduction of oxygen tension promotes enhanced expression of mitogens, including FGF, VEGF, PDGF and their receptors,[27] as well as endothelial cell growth.[28] In addition to factors inducing angiogenesis, the absence of ongoing neovascularisation in normal tissues suggests that the downregulation of normally present angiogenic inhibitors might trigger the starting process of angiogenesis in response to ischaemia. One such potential inhibitor was recently isolated from porcine myocardium and was shown to suppress endothelial cell proliferation *in vitro*.[29]

Members of the HBGF family – including FGF and VEGF – have been tested in the treatment of myocardial ischaemia. In one of the first studies,[30] 2 intracoronary injections of FGF-2 (basic) were given immediately following induction of acute myocardial infarction in dogs. Examination of the hearts 2 weeks later demonstrated a reduction in the infarct size as well as an increase in the number of capillaries and arterioles in the FGF-2–treated animals. Another study of intracoronary injection of FGF-2 in pigs with acute myocardial infarction also demonstrated increased neovascularisation in the treated animals, but failed to show any effect on left ventricular function.[31]

Important benefits have also been obtained in models of chronic myocardial ischaemia treated with HBGF.[32-36] Unlike the studies in acute ischaemia, in which the growth factor was delivered only by intracoronary injections, growth factors have been administered to animals with chronic ischaemia using a variety of techniques that permit sustained delivery; both extravascular and intravascular approaches have been tested.[34,37,38] Administration of FGF-1 and FGF-2 has been reported to induce angiogenesis in the chronically ischaemic porcine myocardium sufficient to improve myocardial perfusion and contractility, reduce infarct size and normalise endothelium-dependent vascular reactivity.[30,31,35,39] In addition, viral-mediated gene transfer has recently been investigated as a method of delivery of angiogenic growth factors in an animal model of chronic ischaemia. This study[32] tested FGF-5 administered by adenoviral-mediated gene transfer, and increased perfusion in the ischaemic myocardium was found as well as increased numbers of capillaries in both normal and ischaemic tissue areas. As with FGF, long-term intracoronary or extracoronary infusion of VEGF resulted in a significant improvement in coronary flow and function of the compromised myocardium.[35,40,41]

In addition to studies in acute and chronic myocardial ischaemia, the angiogenic potency of both FGF and VEGF has been tested in models of peripheral limb ischaemia.[42-44] Injections of FGF-2 or VEGF as well as transfection of DNA encoding VEGF resulted in improved collateral flow and function in the compromised limbs.[42,43] Experimental application of modified fibrin glue with FGF-1 between the descending aorta and the myocardium of the left ventricle resulted in initiating site-directed formation of new blood vessel structures to the heart.[37,38] A more recent study showed that in rats with myocardial ischaemia followed by creation of transmural channels (similar to the principle of transmyocardial laser revascularisation) a significant angiogenic response, in terms of elevated expression of FGF, TGF and VEGF, occurred.[45]

3. Angiogenic Therapy in Humans

On the basis of the experimental research elucidating the efficacy of neo-angiogenesis mediated or initiated by growth factors, especially FGF and VEGF, the first attempts have recently been made to treat patients with coronary or peripheral vascular disease with angiogenic growth factors.[24-26]

Isner et al.[24] demonstrated angiographic and histological evidence of angiogenesis after intra-arterial gene transfer of naked plasmid DNA encoding human VEGF in a patient with critical limb ischaemia. In 1998, Isner's group (Baumgartner et al.[25]) presented the results of intramuscular phVEGF$_{165}$ gene transfer performed in an initial phase I clinical trial comprising 9 patients with 10 critically ischaemic limbs.[25]

Our group reported in 1998 the first angiogenic therapy of human coronary heart disease.[26] Following production and high-grade purification of recombinant human FGF-1 in laboratory research, we directed special attention to careful exclusion of any adverse effects of FGF-1, especially with respect to oncogenity and pyrogenicity. After extensive experimental testing of FGF-1 *in vitro* and *in vivo* we performed a randomised controlled clinical trial with 40 patients. In 20 patients with 3-vessel coronary artery disease who underwent bypass surgery, FGF-1 was injected directly into the myocardium close to the left anterior descending coronary artery and distal to its anastomosis with the internal mammary artery. Transfemoral intra-arterial digital subtraction angiography 12 weeks later showed coronary artery neovascularisation extending out from the area of FGF-1 injection. Stenoses or occlusions distal to the anastomosis were bridged by a *de novo* capillary net, resulting in a 3-fold increase in the local blood supply of the FGF-1 injection sites (figure 1). This was similar to the neovascularisation we observed in rat hearts injected with FGF-1, where histological sections of rat myocardium showed a 3-fold increase in microvessel density. In 20 control patients undergoing similar coronary artery bypass surgery in whom inactivated FGF-1 was injected, there was no evidence of myocardial neovascularisation on the 12-week angiograms. Additionally, the left ventricular function estimated by echography 3 years later showed a significantly better ejection fraction in the FGF-1–treated group in comparison with the control group.

In a preliminary study of 8 patients, Sellke et al.[46] implanted heparin-alginate devices, each containing either 1 or 10μg of FGF-2 (basic), in the epicardial fat of multiple regions of the heart during the bypass operation. At 3 months after the operation, 7 patients had improved or similar left ventricular ejection fraction compared with preoperatively and 3 patients had clear enhancement of perfusion to the unrevascularised myocardium as demonstrated by post-operative myocardial perfusion scanning.

The following differences exist between the procedures of Isner et al.[24,25] and those of our group.[26] In our study we: (i) used FGF-1 as angiogenic growth factor (rather than VEGF); (ii) used the angiogenic growth factor directly (rather than gene transfer of plasmid DNA encoding the growth factor); and (iii) applied the angiogenic growth factor in close proximity to the tissue area to be treated (rather than intra-arterial or intramuscular application). Thus, our procedure does not require the incorporation of DNA into the nucleus of the cells of the recipient. Consequently, we believe that our method has the benefits of simplicity, predictability of dose and restriction of the effect of the angiogenic growth factor. With any kind of systemic application (or distribution) of the angiogenic growth factor some adverse effects may appear. The limited clinical experience with plasmid-mediated VEGF gene therapy has already revealed exacerbation or initiation of local oedema, substantial systemic hypotension or the risk of exacerbation of atherosclerotic plaque neovascularisation.[47,48]

All gene therapy designed to encourage local angiogenesis carries the theoretical risk that pathological angiogenesis at a remote site could be stimulated, for example ocular or tumour

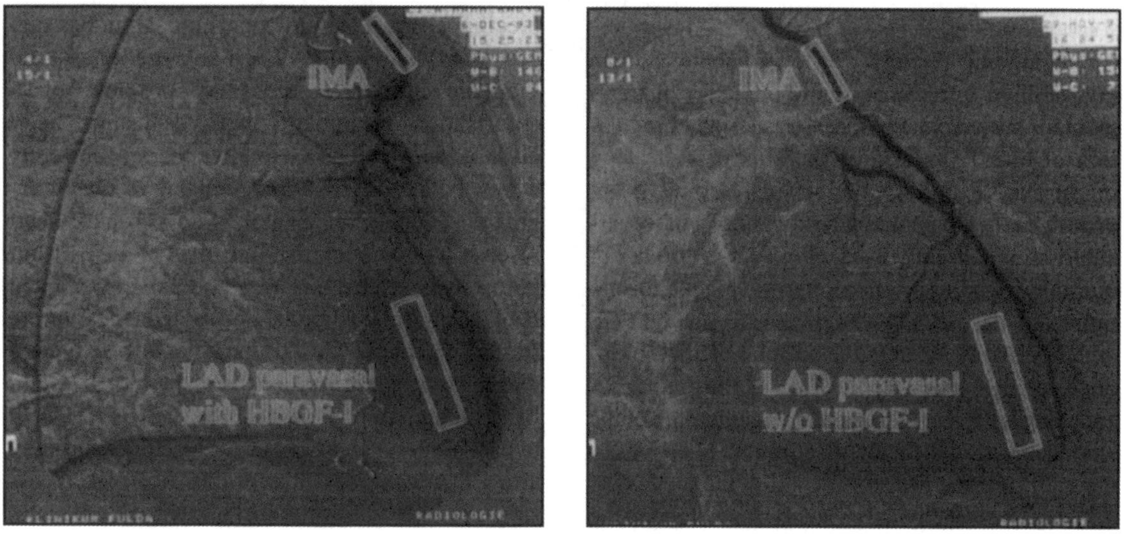

Fig. 1. Angiogenesis induced in the human heart by application of fibroblast growth factor-1 (FGF-1). Neovascularisation was assessed quantitatively by grey value analysis of comparable regions of interest of the angiogram.
Left: patient with FGF-1 (here denoted as 'HBGF-I') application; **right:** control patient without FGF-1 application. **IMA** = internal mammary artery; **LAD** = left anterior descending coronary artery.

angiogenesis. However, in studies of mice bearing dormant microscopic lung metastases, repeated systemic injections of either FGF-2 (basic FGF) or VEGF did not stimulate angiogenesis in these lesions or stimulate tumour growth.[23,48] Furthermore, corneal neovascularisation induced in mice by implantation of a sustained-release pellet of FGF-2 was not enhanced by systemic administration of FGF-2 or VEGF.[48]

Before considering the use of FGF-1 on human patients, our group was able to exclude any tumour-inducing or tumour-stimulating effect of FGF-1 by using *in vitro* assays as well as numerous animal experiments with different species.[26,49-51] No pyrogenic adverse effects of FGF-1 were found.[50] During this research, neither an increase in the rate of growth of a tumour nor an increase in its grading of malignancy were observed to follow the administration of FGF-1.[50] This may be most readily explained by the specific binding of the factor to the high-affinity receptor system on the endothelial cell membrane, and by the absence of hypoxia or ischaemia as triggers for the activation of the angiogenic potential of growth factors.

4. Conclusions

Angiogenic therapy of the ischaemic human myocardium introduces a new modality of treatment for coronary heart disease in terms of regulation of blood vessel growth. This new strategy might evolve into an important alternative approach to the mechanical procedures of revascularisation currently used. However, a number of questions remain. Is atherosclerotic plaque formation really dependent on angiogenesis (i.e. on FGF and/or VEGF)? What is the optimal method to induce angiogenesis – application of plasmid DNA encoding VEGF or FGF, or direct application of the angiogenic growth factor? In addition, questions of the optimal route of administration, the method of delivery and toxicity will need to be resolved in the future. There is also a question of whether this kind of neovascularisation will work in cases of totally diffuse coronary atherosclerosis involving the proximal segments of the main coronary arteries. From the experience of our group,[26,51] it seems to be important that there exists a free-feeding proximal segment of the coronary arteries with which the newly grown vascular structures are connected before distributing into the periphery of the originally obstructed vascular bed. Finally, the question of the best angiogenic growth factor or combination of growth factors in terms of angiogenic efficacy, specificity of directed angiogenesis and minimised adverse effects has to be examined.

Further clinical studies on therapeutic induction of neo-angiogenesis in patients with coronary heart disease need to define specific outcomes in terms of: (i) well-defined clinical end-points, for example death, presence of angina and exercise tolerance; (ii) angiographic end-points, such as quantification of new vessels or collaterals and assessment of coronary blood flow; and (iii) functional end-points, for example assessment of myocardial perfusion by perfusion scanning or magnetic resonance imaging techniques and of global and regional left ventricular function at rest and during exercise.

However, promotion of neovascularisation in patients with ischaemic cardiovascular disease has many attractive features; the data available from preclinical as well as the recent clinical studies suggest that the induction of neo-angiogenesis by angiogenic growth factors may provide revascularisation in patients with ischaemic heart disease for whom no alternative therapy currently exists. Following the first promising results of angiogenic therapy of patients with coronary heart disease by local application of FGF-1,[26,51] our group suggests that this new modality of treatment may become an additional option in the near future for those patients who: (i) have the diffuse type of coronary artery disease not amenable to established interventional procedures such as PTCA or bypass surgery; and/or (ii) have proximal coronary artery lesions (accessible for PTCA and/or bypass surgery) and additional distal stenoses or occlusions of the coronary vascular bed not accessible for PTCA and/or bypass surgery. In these conditions, angiogenic therapy by intramyocardial injection of angiogenic growth factors, such as FGF-1, could serve as an adjunct to routine bypass surgery for coronary heart disease.

Acknowledgements

I would like to thank Mrs S. Faulstich for her assistance in preparation of this manuscript and her technical support.

References

1. Loop FD. Coronary artery surgery: the end of the beginning. Eur J Cardiothorac Surg 1998; 14: 554-71
2. Folkman J, Klagsbrun M. Angiogenic factors. Science 1987; 235: 442-7
3. Folkman J, Shing Y. Angiogenesis. J Biol Chem 1992; 267: 10931-4
4. Folkman J. Clinical applications of research on angiogenesis. N Engl J Med 1995; 333: 1757-63
5. Burgess WH, Mehrman T, Friesel R, et al. Multiple forms of endothelial cell growth factor. Rapid isolation and biological and chemical characterization. J Biol Chem 1985; 260: 11389-92
6. Thomas KA. Vascular endothelial growth factor, a potent and selective angiogenetic agent. J Biol Chem 1996; 271: 603-6
7. Thompson JA, Haudenschild CC, Anderson KD, et al. Heparin-binding growth factor induces the formation of organoid neovascular structures *in vivo*. Proc Natl Acad Sci U S A 1989; 86: 7928-32
8. Dvorak HF, Brown LF, Detmar M, et al. Vascular permeability factor/vascular endothelial growth factor, micro-vascular hyperpermeability and angiogenesis. Am J Pathol 1995; 146: 1029-39
9. Friesel R, Burgess WH, Mehrman T, et al. The characterization of the receptor for endothelial cell growth factor by covalent ligand attachment. J Biol Chem 1986; 261: 7581-4
10. Ware JA, Simons M. Angiogenesis in ischemic heart disease. Nature Med 1997; 3: 158-64

11. Slavin J. Fibroblast growth factors: at the heart of angiogenesis. Cell Biol In 1995; 19: 431-44
12. Kuwabara K, Ogawa S, Matsumoto M, et al. Hypoxia-mediated induction of acidic/basic fibroblast growth factor and platelet-derived growth factor in mononuclear phagocytes stimulates growth of hypoxic endothelial cells. Proc Natl Acad Sci U S A 1995; 92: 4606-10
13. Shweiki D, Itin A, Soffer D, et al. Vascular endothelial growth factor induced by hypoxia may mediate hypoxia-initiated angiogenesis. Nature 1992; 359: 843-5
14. Ferrara N, Carrer-Moore K, Chen H, et al. Heterozygous embryonic lethality induced by targeted inactivation of the VEGF gene. Nature 1996; 380: 439-42
15. Folkman J. Tumor angiogenesis: therapeutic implications. N Engl J Med 1971; 285: 1182-6
16. Gimbrone MA Jr, Cotran RS, Folkman J. Endothelial regeneration and turnover: studies with human endothelial cell cultures. Ser Haematol 1973; 6: 453-5
17. Shing Y, Folkman J, Sullivan R, et al. Heparin affinity: purification of a tumor-derived capillary endothelial cell growth factor. Science 1984; 223: 1296-8
18. Maciag T, Mehrman T, Friesel R, et al. Heparin binds endothelial cell growth factor, the principal mitogen in the bovine brain. Science 1984; 225: 932-5
19. Baird A, Bohlen P, Esch F, et al. Acidic fibroblast growth factor (FGF) from bovine brain: amino-terminal sequence and comparison with basic FGF. EMBO J 1985; 4 (8): 1951-6
20. Taylor S, Folkman J. Protamine is an inhibitor of angiogenesis. Nature 1982; 297: 307-12
21. Crum R, Szabo S, Folkman J. A new class of steroids inhibits angiogenesis in the presence of heparin or a heparin fragment. Science 1985; 230: 1375-8
22. White CW, Sondheimer HM, Crouch EC, et al. Treatment of pulmonary hemangiomatosis with recombinant interferon alfa–2a. N Engl J Med 1989; 320: 1197-200
23. Sorelle R. Two sides of the same coin. Circulation 1998; 98: 383-4
24. Isner JM, Pieczek A, Schainfeld R, et al. Clinical evidence of angiogenesis after arterial gene transfer of ph $VEGF_{165}$ in patient with ischemic limb. Lancet 1996; 348: 370-4
25. Baumgartner J, Pieczek A, Manor O, et al. Constitutive expression of ph $VEGF_{165}$ after intramuscular gene transfer promotes collateral vessel development in patients with critical limb ischemia. Circulation 1998; 97: 1114-23
26. Schumacher B, Pecher P, von Specht BU, et al. Induction of neoangiogenesis in ischemic myocardium by human growth factors. First clinical results of a new treatment of coronary heart disease. Circulation 1998; 97 (7): 645-50
27. Tuder RM, Flook BE, Voelkel NF. Increased gene expression for VEGF and the VEGF receptors KDR/Flk and Flt in lungs exposed to acute or to chronic hypoxia. Modulation of gene expression by nitric oxide. J Clin Invest 1995; 95: 1798-807
28. Nomura M, Yamagishi S, Havada S, et al. Possible participation of autocrine and paracrine vascular endothelial growth factors in hypoxia-induced proliferation of endothelial cells and pericytes. J Biol Chem 1995; 270: 28316-24
29. Westernacher D, Schaper W. A novel heart derived inhibitor of vascular cell proliferation. Purification and biological activity. J Mol Cell Cardiol 1995; 27: 1535-43
30. Yanagisawa-Miwa A, Uchida Y, Nakamura F, et al. Salvage of infarcted myocardium by angiogenic action of basic fibroblast growth factor. Science 1992: 257: 1401-3
31. Battler A, Scheinowitz M, Bor A, et al. Intracoronary injection of basic fibroblast growth factor enhances angiogenesis in infarcted swine myocardium. J Am Coll Cardiol 1993; 22: 2001-6
32. Giordano FJ, Ping P, McKirnan MD, et al. Intracoronary transfer of fibroblast growth factor-5 increases blood flow and contractile function in an ischemic region of the heart. Nature Med 1996; 2: 534-9
33. Lazarous DF, Scheinowitz M, Shou M, et al. Effects of chronic systemic administration of basic fibroblast growth factor on collateral development in the canine heart. Circulation 1995; 91: 145-53
34. Unger EF, Banai S, Shou M, et al. Basic fibroblast growth factor enhances myocardial collateral flow in a canine model. Am J Physiol 1994; 266: 1588-95
35. Harada K, Grossman W, Friedman M, et al. Basic fibroblast growth factor improves myocardial function in chronically ischemic porcine hearts. J Clin Invest 1994; 94: 623-30
36. Banai S, Jaklitsch MT, Casscells W, et al. Effects of acidic fibroblast growth factor on normal and ischemic myocardium. Circulation Res 1991; 69: 76-85
37. Fasol R, Schumacher B, Schlaudraff K, et al. Experimental use of a modified fibrin-glue to induce site-directed angiogenesis from the aorta to the heart. J Thorac Cardiovasc Surg 1994; 107 (6): 1432-9
38. Schlaudraff K, Schumacher B, von Specht BU, et al. Growth of 'new' coronary vascular structures by angiogenetic growth factor. Eur J Cardiothorac Surg 1993; 7 (12): 637-44
39. Sellke FW, Wang SY, Stamler A, et al. Angiogenesis induced by acidic fibroblast growth factor as an alternative method of revascularization for chronic myocardial ischemia. Surgery 1996; 120: 182-8
40. Pearlman JD, Hibberd MG, Chuang ML, et al. Magnetic resonance mapping demonstrates benefits of VEGF-induced myocardial angiogenesis. Nature Med 1995; 1: 1085-9
41. Banai S, Jaklitsch MT, Shou M, et al. Angiogenic-induced enhancement of collateral flow to ischemic myocardium by vascular endothelial growth factor in dogs. Circulation 1994; 89: 2183-9
42. Baffour R, Berman J, Garb JL, et al. Enhanced angiogenesis and growth of collaterals by in vivo administration of recombinant basic fibroblast growth factor in a rabbit model of acute lower limb ischemia: dose-response effect of basic fibroblast growth factor. J Vasc Surg 1992; 16: 181-91
43. Mack CA, Magovern CJ, Budenbender KT, et al. Salvage angiogenesis induced by adenovirus-mediated gene transfer of vascular endothelial growth factor protects against ischemic vascular occlusion. J Vasc Surg 1998; 27: 699-709
44. Takeshita S. Zheng LP, Brogi E, et al. Therapeutic angiogenesis. Single intraarterial bolus of vascular endothelial growth factor augments revascularization in a rabbit ischemic hind limb model. J Clin Invest 1994; 93: 662-70

45. Pelletier MP, Giaid A, Sivaraman S, et al. Angiogenesis and growth factor expression in a model of transmyocardial revascularization. Ann Thorac Surg 1998; 66: 12-8
46. Sellke FW, Laham RJ, Edelman R, et al. Therapeutic angiogenesis with basic fibroblast growth factor: technique and early results. Ann Thorac Surg 1998; 65: 1540-4
47. Kuzuya M, Satake S, Esaki T, et al. Induction of angiogenesis by smooth muscle cell-derived factor: possible role in neovascularization in atherosclerotic plaque. J Cell Physiol 1995; 164: 658-67
48. Folkman J. Therapeutic angiogenesis in ischemic limbs [editorial]. Circulation 1998; 97: 1108-10
49. Folkman J. Angiogenic therapy of the human heart [editorial]. Circulation 1998; 97 (7): 628-9
50. Schumacher B, von Specht BU, Haberstroh J, et al. The stimulation of neo-angiogenesis in the ischemic heart by the human growth factor FGF. J Cardiovasc Surg 1998; 39: 445-53
51. Schumacher B, Stegmann T, Pecher P. The stimulation of neoangiogenesis in the ischemic human heart by the growth factor FGF: first clinical results. J Cardiovasc Surg 1998; 39 (6): 783-9

Correspondence: Prof. Dr *Thomas J. Stegmann*, Department of Thoracic and Cardiovascular Surgery, Fulda Medical Center, Pacelliallee 4, 36043 Fulda, Germany.
E-mail: heart.stegmann@klinikum-fulda.de